Palliative Care Consultations in Haemato-oncology

Series information

Series editors

Sara Booth
Macmillan Consultant in Palliative Medicine,
Addenbrooke's Palliative Care Service,
Cambridge,
UK

Eduardo Bruera
Professor,
Chair, Department of Palliative Care & Rehabilitation Medicine,
University of Texas M.D. Anderson Cancer Center,
Houston, TX,
USA

Advisory editor

Jenny Craig
Consultant Haematologist,
Addenbrooke's Palliative Care Team,
Cambridge,
UK

Palliative Care Consultations in Haemato-oncology

Sara Booth

Macmillan Consultant in Palliative Medicine,
Addenbrooke's Palliative Care Service,
Cambridge, UK

Eduardo Bruera

Professor,
Chair, Department of Palliative Care & Rehabilitation
Medicine,
University of Texas M.D. Anderson Cancer Center,
Houston, TX, USA

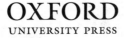

OXFORD

UNIVERSITY PRESS

OXFORD
UNIVERSITY PRESS

Great Clarendon Street, Oxford OX2 6DP

Oxford University Press is a department of the University of Oxford.
It furthers the University's objective of excellence in research, scholarship,
and education by publishing worldwide in

Oxford New York

Auckland Bangkok Buenos Aires Cape Town Chennai
Dar es Salaam Delhi Hong Kong Istanbul Karachi Kolkata
Kuala Lumpur Madrid Melbourne Mexico City Mumbai Nairobi
São Paulo Shanghai Taipei Tokyo Toronto

Oxford is a registered trade mark of Oxford University Press
in the UK and in certain other countries

Published in the United States
by Oxford University Press Inc., New York

© Oxford University Press, 2003

A catalogue record for this title is available from the British Library

ISBN 0 19 852808 6

10 9 8 7 6 5 4 3 2 1

Typeset by Newgen Imaging Systems (P) Ltd., Chennai, India
Printed in Great Britain
on acid-free paper by
Biddles Ltd, Guildford & King's Lynn

Palliative Care Consultations Series Foreword

Professor M A Richards
National Cancer Director, England

Despite the significant advances in diagnosis and treatment that have been made in recent decades, cancer remains a major cause of death in all developed countries. It is therefore essential that all health professionals who provide direct care for cancer patients should be aware of what can be done to alleviate suffering.

Major progress has been made over the past thirty years or so in the relief of physical symptoms and in approaches to the delivery of psychological, social, and spiritual care for cancer patients and their families and carers. However, the problems of providing holistic care should not be underestimated. This is particularly the case in busy acute general hospitals and cancer centres. The physical environment may not be conducive to the care of a dying patient. Staff may have difficulty recognizing the point at which radical interventions are no longer in a patient's best interests, when the emphasis should change to care with palliative intent.

Progress in the treatment of cancer has also led to many patients who, although incurable, live for years with their illness. They may have repeated courses of treatment and some will have a significant burden of symptoms which must be optimally controlled.

One of the most important developments in recent years has been the recognition of the benefits of a multidisciplinary or multiprofessional approach to cancer care. Physicians, surgeons, radiologists, haematologists, pathologists, oncologists, palliative care specialists, nurse specialists, and a wide range of other health professionals all have major contributions to make. These specialists need to work together in teams.

One of the prerequisites for effective teamwork is that individual members should recognize the contribution that others can make. The *Palliative Care Consultations* series should help to make this a reality. The editors are to be congratulated in bringing together distinguished cancer and palliative care specialists from all parts of the world. Individual volumes focus predominantly on the problems faced by patients with a particular type of cancer (e.g. breast or lung) or groups of cancers (e.g. haematological malignancies or gynaecological cancers). The chapters of each volume set out what can be achieved using anticancer treatments and through the delivery of palliative care.

I warmly welcome the series and I believe the individual volumes will prove valuable to a wide range of clinicians involved in the delivery of high quality care.

Preface

This book forms part of a series dedicated to the palliative care of patients in the acute setting. Cancer medicine and palliative care have both changed enormously in recent years. Cancer has become a chronic illness for all but those with the most advanced disease at diagnosis. Patients undergo more and more intensive treatments with sophisticated supportive care and multiple interventions with large numbers of doctors, nurses, and other professionals (clinical and non-clinical) involved in their care.

Patients who have haematological malignancy often undergo the most rigorous treatments often requiring long in-patient stays at tertiary referral centres far removed from friends, families, and everyday life. They embark on this treatment regimen precipitously and if their treatment is unsuccessful their prognosis may be very short indeed. They may also be disfigured and emotionally distressed by the demands of the intensive therapy and even those who are cured will undergo a period of painful and difficult treatment with many adverse effects, some of which are long-term. The treatment for some malignancies is palliative, although aggressive, from diagnosis and patients may live with a heavy burden of symptoms if these are not controlled.

Palliative care teams working in acute hospitals are often involved both with those who are curable and those who are not. It is more and more common for supportive care (including palliative care) to be standard right from the beginning of in-patient treatment. Haematology units tend to attract very dedicated staff who work hard to see patients through their demanding treatments and may feel desperately distressed when things are going wrong. There is often a difficult transition into palliative care, which patients find traumatic and they may often feel abandoned. Sometimes death follows quickly after the withdrawal of chemotherapy. Many of the patients are very young and had the expectation of long life, many have children, and most are in work and have to balance this with their treatment. These circumstances alone can impose enormous strains and tensions on both patients and staff dealing with the palliation of haematological malignancy.

Patients can lose touch with their family physicians and community primary care teams: this easily happens as the patient and family often spend most of their time in or at the hospital. It is vitally important that the hospital teams keep the general practitioner/family physician up to date with what is happening – whether the news be good or bad.

It is now increasingly understood that excellent palliative care may involve treatment with blood and blood products, intravenous drugs, and other interventions once thought alien to giving holistic patient-centred care. Sometimes these treatments are most appropriately given on the acute unit and sometimes in the specialist palliative care unit. In some areas it is possible to give intravenous therapies in the patient's home. This would have been an unusual idea 10 years ago. This volume addresses these changes. It is essential that the haematology and the palliative care teams work in an integrated way so that a 'precipitous drop' into palliative care is avoided when and if things go badly. Other patients need palliation from the time of diagnosis but the expertise of the haematologist is vital if the patient is to have optimal care.

There are many excellent textbooks on general palliative care and this series does not cover the same ground. This book is intended to give the reader the science and practice of hospital palliative care – it is designed to be reached for before (or during) a day on the wards or in out-patients or even on a domiciliary visit. It is intended to give practical advice on difficult symptom control problems which are seen very commonly in hospital palliative care but more rarely for clinicians practising in the hospice or community. We think it will be of use not only to palliative care physicians, specialist nurses, and others in palliative care in the hospital or hospice but also to doctors, nurses, and others who specialize in haematology. Although it is centred on hospital palliative care it is likely to be helpful to anyone caring for a patient with haematological malignancy.

We are grateful to all our contributors for their expertise and commitment. Dr Jenny Craig has been a superb advisory editor. This is the first volume in a series and we were learning too, adding some chapters reviewing the basics of symptom control at the request of various haematologists and one on the basics of bone marrow transplantation when it was clear that this subject was difficult for some palliative care physicians.

We hope that you enjoy reading and using this book as much as we have enjoyed preparing it.

SB
EB
May 2003

Contents

Contributors

Cathy Alban-Jones
Clinical Nurse Specialist,
Addenbrooke's Palliative Care Team,
Cambridge, UK

Pia Amsler
Specialist Registrar in Palliative
Medicine, Addenbrooke's Hospital,
Cambridge, UK

Dr Wale Atoyebi
Department of Haematology,
John Radcliffe Hospital,
Oxford, UK

Helen Balsdon
Haematology Senior Nurse,
Addenbrooke's Hospital,
Cambridge, UK

Kristian Bowles
SpR in Haematology
Department of Haematology,
Norfolk and Norwich Hospital,
Norwich, UK

Susan Closs
Ty Olwen Hospice,
Morriston Hospital,
Swansea, UK

Jenny I. O. Craig
Consultant Haematologist,
Addenbrookes Hospital,
Cambridge, UK

Pablo Desmery
Chief of Intensive Care Unit,
'Angélica Ocampo' Hospitalisation
and Clinical Research Center,
Fundaleu, Buenos Aires, Argentina

María Cecilia Dignani
'Angélica Ocampo' Hospitalisation
and Clinical Research Center,
Fundaleu,
Buenos Aires, Argentina

Baroness Finlay of Llandaff
Vice Dean,
School of Medicine, University of
Wales School of Medicine, and
Section of Palliative Medicine,
Velindre NHS Trust,
Cardiff, UK

Fiona Hicks
Consultant in Palliative Medicine
Leeds Teaching Hospitals Trust, UK

Beverley Hunt
Consultant Haematologist
Department of Haematology,
St Thomas' Hospital,
London, UK

David Jeffrey
Macmillan Consultant in
Palliative Medicine,
Gloucestershire Oncology Centre,
General Hospital,
Cheltenham, UK

Tim Littlewood
Consultant Haematologist,
John Radcliffe Hospital,
Oxford, UK

Robert Marcus
Consultant Haematologist,
Addenbrookes Hospital,
Cambridge, UK

Mary Miller
Consultant in Palliative Medicine,
Sir Michael Sobell House,
Churchill Hospital,
Oxford, UK

Lorraine Moth
Communinty Nurse,
Arthur Rank House,
Cambridge, UK

Ghulam Mufti
Department of Haematology,
Guy's, King's and Thomas'
School of Medicine,
London, UK

Simon Noble
SpR in Palliative Medicine,
University Hospital Wales,
Cardiff,
Wales, UK

Ray Owen
Palliative Care Team,
Gloucester Royal Hospital,
Gloucester, UK

Santiago Pavlovsky
Medical Director,
'Angélica Ocampo' Hospitalisation
and Clinical Research Center,
Fundaleu,
Buenos Aires, Argentina

Paul Perkins
Specialist Registrar in Palliative
Medicine,
Ty Olwen Hospice,
Morriston Hospital,
Swausea, UK

Russell K. Portenoy
Chairman,
Department of Pain Medicine and
Palliative Care,
Beth Israel Medical Center,
New York, New York
and
Professor of Neurology,
Albert Einstein College of Medicine,
Bronx, New York, USA

Kavita Raj
Guy's, King's and Thomas' School of
Medicine,
London, UK

Anna Spathis
Specialist Registrar in Palliative
Medicine,
Addenbrooke's Hospital,
Cambridge, UK

Robert Twycross
Macmillan Clinical Reader in
Palliative Medicine,
Sir Michael Sobell House,
Churchill Hospital, Oxford, UK

Annette Vielhaber
Department of Pain Medicine and
Palliative Care,
Beth Israel Medical Center, New York,
New York, USA

Rosemary Wade
St Nicholas Hospice,
Bury St Edmunds, UK

Chapter 1

Management of myeloma

Jenny I. O. Craig

Multiple myeloma is a clonal B cell disorder with an incidence of 4/100 000 in UK. It is a disease of the elderly with a median age at presentation of 69 years and a median survival of 3 years from diagnosis. The clinical features of myeloma result from the three salient features of the disease:

(1) a malignant proliferation of plasma cells in the bone marrow

(2) the production by the malignant plasma cells of a monoclonal immunoglobulin (m protein, m band, or paraprotein) detectable in blood and/or immunoglobulin light chains (Bence Jones protein) in the urine

(3) bony destruction with lytic lesions and osteoporosis.

The disease is staged by estimating the myeloma mass using paraprotein levels, clinical parameters, and bone disease, as shown in Table 1.1, and gives an indicator of survival. Newer methods of disease assessment include cytogenetic analysis for monosomy 13 or deletion of chromosome 13 (poor prognostic features); magnetic resonance imaging of bones may give further useful information about prognosis and response to therapy.

Pathogenesis

Malignant plasma cells are clonal, terminally differentiated B cells with a low proliferative index. The myeloma 'stem cell' or precursor cell in the malignant clone is a memory B cell or plasmablast from lymphoid tissues. This circulates and homes to the bone marrow, binding to stromal cells via adhesion molecules. The interaction between plasma cells and the bone marrow micro-environment is important, promoting growth and survival of myeloma cells. For example, interleukin-6 (IL-6) secretion by the stromal cell, which stimulates plasma cell proliferation, is stimulated by myeloma cell adhesion. Interleukin-6 secretion is further up regulated by cytokines (tumour necrosis factor alpha (TNF-α), TGF-β and VEGF) from myeloma plasma cells. These cytokines also increase myeloma cell growth, protect against drug induced apoptosis, augment binding to the stroma, and stimulate angiogenesis in the

Table 1.1 Durie Salmon staging of myeloma

Stage		Myeloma mass (estimated numbers of plasma cells)	Median survival
I	All of: Hb >10 g/dl, normal bone structure, normal calcium, IgG < 50 g/l or IgA <30 g/l or Bence Jones protein <4 g/24 h	$<0.6 \times 10^{12}/m^2$	72 months
II	Neither stage I or III	$0.6–1.2 \times 10^{12}/m^2$	56 months
III	One of: Hb <8.5 g/dl, raised calcium >3 mmol/l advanced bone disease (>3 lytic bone lesions) IgG >70 g/dl, or IgA >50 g/dl or Bence Jones protein >12 g/24 h	$>1.2 \times 10^{12}/m^2$	24 months
	In addition, subdivided to: (a) normal renal function; (b) abnormal renal function		

bone marrow micro-environment, thus supporting the survival of this disease. Accumulation of plasma cells in the marrow leads to bone marrow failure with anaemia, thrombocytopenia and leukopenia.

The secretion of a monoclonal immunoglobulin (Ig) is often associated with suppression of normal immunoglobulins (immunoparesis) causing susceptibility to infection. Accumulation of the paraprotein can cause hyperviscosity or lead to deposition of light chains in the kidneys contributing to renal failure. The incidence of M protein types in myeloma is shown in Table 1.2.

Bone disease in myeloma

Bone disease in myeloma is a consequence of bone loss and causes considerable morbidity from pain, pathological fractures, vertebral collapse, and hypercalcaemia. Bone loss in myeloma is a consequence of increased bone resorption and reduced bone formation.

Increased bone resorption results from stimulation of bone resorbing cells (osteoclasts) by soluble factors from the myeloma cells and the bone marrow

Table 1.2 The incidence of M-band
(paraprotein) types in myeloma

IgG	53%
IgA	25%
Light chains only	17%
IgD	2%
IgE	Rare
Bi-clonal	3%
Non-secretory	<1%

micro-environment. These osteoclast-activating factors (OAF) include TNF-β and IL-1β. More recently it has been shown that TNF-α, which stimulates the release of NFκB (an inducer of bone resorption), plays a major role in myeloma bone loss. These factors act through a final common pathway to stimulate bone resorption, which is thought to include the receptor RANK on the surface of osteoclasts and its ligand RANKL that can be found on marrow stromal cells, osteoblasts and myeloma cells. An inhibitor molecule called osteoprotegrin (OPG) has been discovered that binds RANKL, preventing the binding of RANKL to RANK and hence inhibits bone loss. The amount of bone loss depends upon the balance between OPG and RANKL. This system is under investigation as a therapeutic target in myeloma bone disease.

Clinical presentation

Myeloma can cause widespread symptoms and therefore patients may present to many different specialties in medicine. The presenting symptoms and signs of myeloma are shown in Table 1.3.

Assessment

The history and examination may reveal symptoms and signs of the presenting features (Table 1.3). Haematological investigations will show a normochromic normocytic anaemia in 60%, rouleaux, a raised ESR and plasma viscosity. In advanced disease there may be neutropenia and thrombocytopenia and, in about 15%, circulating plasma cells. On biochemical testing there will be a raised total protein, reduced serum albumin, and on serum protein electrophoresis, an M-band spike (paraprotein) with reduced background globulins is usually found. The type of monoclonal immunoglobulin is determined by immunoelectrophoresis of serum and/or urine and the paraprotein can be

Table 1.3 Presenting features of myeloma

Common	**Bone pain** (70%), often back pain and vertebral collapse with nerve compression, pathological fractures **Impaired renal function** (50%) **General malaise**, fatigue due to anaemia **Infections** due to bone marrow failure and immune paresis
Less frequent	Hyperviscosity—impaired cerebration, visual deterioration, purpura Hypercalcaemia Spinal cord compression Amyloidosis Cryoglobulinaemia

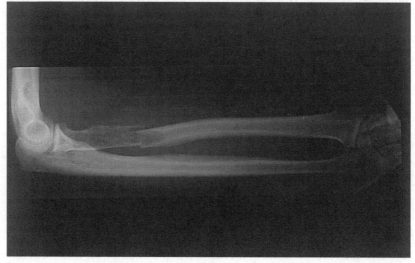

Fig. 1.1 X-ray of forearm showing a pathological fracture of the proximal and of the radius.

quantified for staging and monitoring the progress of disease. Renal failure will result in a raised urea and creatinine and the serum calcium may be elevated.

Bone disease should be assessed by an X-ray skeletal survey. Osteolytic lesions occur in axial skeleton, have regular clear margins, and are symmetrical. The isotope bone scan is usually negative as there is no increase in local bone formation. At presentation, 20% have a normal skeletal survey, 10–15% diffuse osteopenia, and 65% osteopenia and focal lytic lesions. A pathological fracture of the radius is shown in Fig. 1.1 and a plasmacytoma arising from the ileum with marked bone destruction in Fig. 1.2.

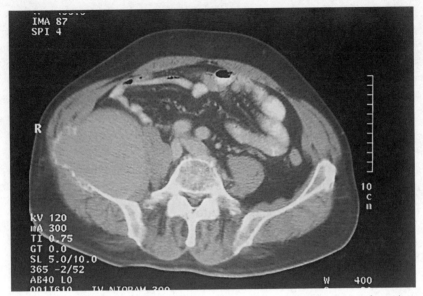

Fig. 1.2 CT scan of pelvis revealing a large soft tissue plasmacytoma arising from the R) ileum.

A bone marrow examination by aspirate and trephine biopsy may show plasma cell infiltration, usually over 15%.

Management

Myeloma is incurable by conventional chemotherapy. Supportive therapy to ensure the best quality of life is of paramount importance. Care of myeloma is multidisciplinary, including general practitioners and community services, haematology, palliative care, renal services, radiotherapists, orthopaedic, neurosurgical and rehabilitation teams, and patients' support groups.

General supportive care

The following supportive measures are important for patients with myeloma.

Hydration

Aiming for an oral fluid intake of at least 3 l/day and the avoidance of nephrotoxic drugs, where possible, is important to optimize renal function.

Pain control

This is paramount (Chapters 8 and 9 give further detail). The type of pain should be assessed and treated appropriately with input from palliative-care services. Bone pain and neuropathic pain as a result of nerve compression are common. Bone pain can be controlled using an analgesic regimen based on the WHO pain ladder, giving paracetamol regularly for mild pain and using opioids for pain of increasing severity. Radiotherapy can give effective local pain relief and orthopedic surgery may be required as treatment or prophylaxis for pathological fractures. Maintaining mobility with the help of physiotherapy support is important to reduce bone loss and maintain quality of life. Neuropathic pain tends to be poorly responsive to opioids but may be controlled by a regimen that includes an anti-convulsant (e.g. gabapentin) or anti-depressant (e.g. amitriptyline) drug, which may be used in combination. Occasionally a nerve block or regional blockade is needed particularly when a patient suffers incident neuropathic pain.

Bisphosphonates (osteoclast inhibitors)

These have been shown to reduce skeletal morbidity, improve quality of life, and reduce the need for surgery and radiotherapy in myeloma bone disease. They may also reduce bony pain in the longer term. A survival advantage has been reported in a subgroup analysis of a study suggesting a disease-modifying role for pamidronate. There is also evidence that patients without overt skeletal disease benefit from bisphosphonate therapy, which may be given intravenously (pamidronate or zoledronate) or orally (clodronate). It is therefore recommended that all patients with myeloma receive long-term bisphosphonate therapy.

Bisphosphonates and hydration should be used in the management of hypercalcaemia.

Infection

Infection should be treated promptly, as myeloma patients are immuno-supressed both as a result of the disease and a consequence of therapy. This may require rapid admission to hospital for intravenous antibiotics in severe sepsis or those undergoing intensive chemotherapy. Patients should be offered influenza vaccine in the community. For some patients with recurrent severe infections, intravenous immunoglobulin replacement may be clinically useful.

Hyperviscosity

In the acute situation, this can be managed by therapeutic plasma exchange until chemotherapy has a chance to take effect.

Anaemia

This is common, occurring in 60% of patients with myeloma. It may improve with treatment of the disease but symptomatic benefit can be gained from careful red cell transfusion, which is generally the mainstay of therapy of anaemia. Care must be taken not to precipitate hyperviscosity symptoms in those with high paraprotein levels.

Erythropoietin (Epo) has been shown to improve haemoglobin levels, reduce transfusion requirements, and improve quality of life in studies of patients with malignancy, including myeloma. Between 50 and 60% of patients with myeloma may respond to Epo but there are no reliable predictors of response. National guidelines recommend that a trial of Epo should be considered in patients with symptomatic anaemia and that it is the treatment of choice for anaemia in patients with myeloma and chronic renal failure.

Spinal cord compression

This may occur as a result of myelomatous destruction of vertebrae or a soft tissue mass in the paravertebral tissues. This is a medical emergency and these patients should be admitted to hospital for investigation by MRI scanning and initial treatment with dexamethasone and radiotherapy.

Renal failure

In myeloma, renal failure is common (in up to 50% at some stage of the disease). It is usually multi-factorial, resulting from light-chain deposition in the kidney (myeloma kidney), dehydration, infection, drugs (especially non steroidal anti-inflammatory drugs), hypercalcaemia, and less often from amyloid, plasma cell infiltration, hyperuricaemia. Many patients can improve with vigorous support, including rehydration, withdrawal of nephrotoxic drugs, treatment of infection, and correction of hypercalcaemia with bisphosphonates. For those with progressive disease, dexamethasone chemotherapy should be used initially until the results of initial supportive therapy are known and a suitable chemotherapy regimen can be instituted if appropriated.

The advice of the renal team should be sought. Dialysis may be required in the acute situation and on a long-term basis.

Initial chemotherapy

Chemotherapy is indicated for symptomatic myeloma usually stage II or III disease, but not for those without evidence of symptoms, bone marrow failure or skeletal lesions. The initial chemotherapy regimen aims to induce a stable response or 'plateau' phase. The choice of drug depends on the patient's age, performance status, and eligibility to undergo a future stem cell transplant.

The mainstay of therapy for patients not planned for stem cell transplant are alkylating agents, either melphalan or cyclophosphamide, with or without steroids. This is usually melphalan at a dose of 6–8 mg/m^2/day for 4–7 days, every 4–6 weeks, which will induce a gradual response in over 50% patients and should be continued until the disease is stable for 3 months. The benefit of the addition of prednisolone is controversial. Melphalan is well tolerated but does cause myelosupression. As its absorption from the gastro-intestinal tract is variable the full blood count requires regular monitoring to establish the dose level. It is excreted via the kidney and should only be used with great caution in renal impairment.

Cyclophosphamide given orally or intravenously gives similar results to melphalan but tends to cause less myelosuppresion. Various combination chemotherapy regimens have been tried but none have shown any advantage over melphalan.

As melphalan is myelotoxic, the combination of vincristine and adriamycin given as a 4 day continuous infusion with oral dexamethasone for 4 days (VAD), which does not damage stem cells, has become the regimen of choice for those planned for stem cell mobilization and transplantation. This induces a rapid response rate of 60–80%, with complete remissions in 10%. It can be given in patients with renal failure. The disadvantages of VAD include the need for a long-term in-dwelling central line, myelosuppression, alopecia, and steroid-related side-effects. The responses are not durable and consolidation, e.g. with a stem cell transplant, is usually given. An oral alternative regimen (idarubicin and dexamethasone, ZDex) seems to give similar results; a randomized comparative trial with VAD is in progress. If chemotherapy is contra-indicated, high dose dexamethasone alone is useful initial treatment, in particular in those with renal failure.

Autologous stem cell transplantation

This may be offered to younger patients under 60 years old to prolong survival further, but not cure, as relapse inevitably occurs. It is reported to increase 5-year event-free (28% versus 10%) and overall survival (52% versus 12%). In patients aged 60 and over, there is no evidence for a survival advantage of autologous transplants. Patients suitable for autologous transplantation, are treated with VAD-type chemotherapy to plateau phase, stem cells are mobilized into the blood, collected by leukapheresis and stored, usually in the vapour phase of liquid nitrogen. The transplant itself involves the administration of conditioning chemotherapy, commonly melphalan 200 mg/m^2, followed by the infusion of stored stem cells. Until the stem cells engraft and peripheral blood counts recover, the patients require intensive support for bone marrow failure and other side-effects of chemotherapy. After high-dose melphalan gastro-intestinal toxicity, often with severe mucositis, is common. In addition to morbidity, autologous peripheral blood stem cell transplantation carries a transplant-related mortality of around 5%. Although most are discharged from hospital within 3–4 weeks, patients generally feel weak and fatigued after transplant. With a gradual increase in activities, most will regain a good quality of life by 3 months after the transplant.

Allogeneic stem cell transplantation

Allogeneic stem cell transplantation from an HLA-identical sibling is the only curative option currently available in myeloma. However, this procedure carries a high transplant-related mortality (20–40%) and risk of relapse post transplant. Because of toxicity, only patients up to the age of 50 years are eligible for consideration of allogeneic transplant and as there is only a one in four chance of a sibling being an HLA identical match, few patients can be considered for this treatment. In those who relapse or have persistent disease after transplant there is evidence that donor lymphocyte infusions exert a 'graft versus myeloma' immune-therapy effect and can induce remission. Low-intensity allografts, where the toxicity of the conditioning regimen is less and which harness the immunotherapy of donor lymphocyte infusions, are currently under investigation and may allow this therapy to be available to an older age group.

Maintenance therapy

There is evidence that interferon-maintenance therapy prolongs the length of plateau phase. However, it has considerable side-effects, in particular flu-like symptoms and malaise, which have a considerable impact on quality of life. This, taken with the less clear benefit on overall survival, tends to limit the use of interferon maintenance.

Management of progressive disease

Myeloma inevitably progresses, and some patients are refractory to initial therapy. The focus of care is to maintain quality of life by controlling disease where possible and to ameliorate symptoms. If relapse occurs early, this carries a poor prognosis, suggesting limited response to further chemotherapy. Further control is more likely in those that have achieved a stable plateau phase for many months. In those suitable for further chemotherapy, about 50% will respond to a second course of oral melphalan. Oral cyclophosphamide is also useful in achieving further control, as is intermittent high-dose dexamethasone. Recently, thalidomide produced responses in about one-third of patients with refractory disease, although higher doses can cause significant side-effects such as somnolence and constipation. In refractory and relapsed patients, the general supportive measures outlined earlier are of paramount importance, in particular good communication between hospital and community to allow full utilization of support networks available to help the patients and their family.

Further reading

Attal, M., Harousseau, J. L., Stoppa, A. M. *et al.* (1996). A prospective randomised trial of autologous transplantation and chemotherapy in multiple myeloma. *N Engl J Med* **335**: 91–7.

Barlogie, B., Desikan, R., Eddlemon, P. *et al.* (2001). Extended survival in advanced and refractory multiple myeloma after single-agent thalidomide: identification of prognostic factors in a phase 2 study of 169 patients. *Blood* **98**(2): 492–4.

Berenson, J. R., Lichtenstein, A., Porter, L. *et al.* (1996). Efficacy of pamidronate in reducing skeletal events in patients with advanced multiple myeloma. Myeloma Aredia Study Group. *N Engl J Med* **334**: 488–93.

British Committee for Standards in Haematology (2001). Guidelines in the diagnosis and management of multiple myeloma. *Br J Haematol* **115**: 522–40.

Clark, A. D., Shetty, A., and Soutar, R. (1999). Renal failure and multiple myeloma: pathogenesis and treatment of renal failure and management of underlying myeloma. *Blood Rev* **13**: 79–90.

Dammacco, F., Castoldi, G., and Rodjer, S. (2001). Efficacy of epoetin alfa in the treatment of anaemia of multiple myeloma. *Br J Haematol* **113**: 172–9.

Gahrton, G., Svensson, H., Cavo, M. *et al.* (2001). Progress in allogenic bone marrow and peripheral blood stem cell transplantation for multiple myeloma: a comparison between transplants performed 1983–93 and 1994–98 at European Group for Blood and Marrow Transplantation centres. *Br J Haematol* **113**: 209–16.

Myeloma Trialists' Collaborative Group (1998). Combination chemotherapy versus melphalan plus prednisone as treatment for multiple myeloma: An overview of 6,633 patients from 27 randomised trials. *J Clin Oncol* **16**: 3832–42.

Samson, D., Gaminara, E., Newland, A. *et al.* (1989). Infusion of vincristine and doxorubicin with oral dexamethasone as first-line therapy for multiple myeloma. *Lancet* **2**: 882–5.

Chapter 2

Management of lymphoma

Kristian Bowles and Robert Marcus

Introduction

Background

Lymphoma describes a number of malignant diseases that arise from lymphoid tissues. There are many histological subtypes of lymphoma and one of the most significant advances in the management of lymphoma has been the World Health Organization Classification (Table 2.1). The histological subtype will in part guide treatment and prognosis.

Many patients diagnosed with lymphoma are cured. Of those that die of their disease, some have received initial therapy with curative intent, whilst others present with incurable disease. Patients' symptoms are frequently determined by the distribution of the disease. There is a good evidence-base for the first-line therapies in the management of lymphoma and clinical trials are continuing to improve treatment and outcome. The management of patients in whom first-line therapy has failed is less evidence-based. Bone marrow transplant is increasingly used to prolong survival in patients with relapsed lymphoma. There is great hope that newer treatments, which include monoclonal antibodies, will improve survival for many patients in the future.

Distribution of disease

Most patients with lymphoma present with lymphadenopathy. Clinical examination will detect lymphadenopathy in the neck, axillae, and groins. Intra-abdominal and intra-thoracic presentation may be difficult to diagnose and is usually assessed by radiological imaging (chest X-ray, ultrasound, and computed tomography scanning). The bone marrow and spleen are also commonly infiltrated with the tumour, particularly in low-grade lymphoma. Any organ system may be affected by lymphoma, as lymphoid cells exist in all organs in the body. Extra-nodal lymphoma, affecting sites such as the central nervous system, gut, lung, skin, head, and neck, can produce distressing and troublesome symptoms. Involvement of each organ system provides its own unique problems for the patient, the family, and the medical team.

Table 2.1 Classification of lymphoma: (a) an overview; (b) the detailed WHO classification

(a) Hodgkin's disease (HD)	Classical HD	
	Nodular lymphocyte predominant HD	
Non-Hodgkin's lymphoma	High grade	T cell
		B cell
	Low grade	T cell
		B cell

(b) B-cell neoplasms	T-cell and natural killer cell neoplasms
I. Precursor B-cell neoplasm:	I. Precursor T cell neoplasm:
a. Precursor B-lymphoblastic leukemia/lymphoma	a. Precursor T-lymphoblastic lymphoma/leukaemia
II. Mature (peripheral) B-cell neoplasms	II. Mature (peripheral) T cell and NK-cell neoplasms:
a. B-cell chronic lymphocytic leukaemia/ small lymphocytic lymphoma	a. T cell prolymphocytic leukaemia
b. B-cell prolymphocytic leukaemia	b. T-cell granular lymphocytic leukaemia
c. Lymphoplasmacytic lymphoma	c. Aggressive NK-Cell leukaemia
d. Splenic marginal zone B-cell lymphoma (+/− villous lymphocytes)	d. Adult T cell lymphoma/leukaemia (HTLV1+)
e. Hairy cell leukaemia	e. Extranodal NK/T-cell lymphoma, nasal type
f. Plasma cell myeloma/plasmacytoma	f. Enteropathy-type T-cell lymphoma
g. Extranodal marginal zone B-cell lymphoma of mucosa-associated lymphoid tissue type	g. Hepatosplenic gamma-delta T-cell lymphoma
h. Nodal marginal zone lymphoma of (+/− monocytoid B-cells)	h. Subcutaneous panniculitis-like T-cell lymphoma
i. Follicle center lymphoma, follicular,	i. Mycosis fungoides/Sézary's syndrome
j. Mantle cell lymphoma	j. Anaplastic large cell lymphoma, T/null cell, primary cutaneous type
k. Diffuse large cell B-cell lymphoma ♦ Mediastinal large B-cell lymphoma ♦ Primary effusion lymphoma	k. Peripheral T cell lymphoma, not otherwise characterized
l. Burkitt's lymphoma/Burkitt's cell leukaemia	l. Angioimmunoblastic T cell lymphoma

Table 2.1 (continued)

(b) B-cell neoplasms	T-cell and natural killer cell neoplasms
	m. Anaplastic large cell lymphoma, T/null cell, primary systemic
	Type Hodgkin's lymphoma (Hodgkin's Disease)
	a. Nodular lymphocyte predominance Hodgkin's lymphoma
	b. Classical Hodgkin's lymphoma
	◆ Nodular sclerosis Hodgkin's lymphoma
	◆ Lymphocyte-rich classical Hodgkin's lymphoma
	◆ Mixed cellularity Hodgkin's lymphoma
	◆ Lymphocyte depletion Hodgkin's lymphoma

Many of the symptoms of lymphoma are not related to the distribution of the disease but occur as a systemic effect of the tumour. The commonest systemic symptoms are weight loss, fevers, and drenching sweats, and appear to affect patients with Hodgkin's disease more frequently than those with non-Hodgkin's lymphoma. Itching, which is more commonly associated with Hodgkin's disease, can be very distressing. Other rare systemic complications include hypercalcaemia and paraneoplastic neurological syndromes.

Histological subtypes of lymphoma

Lymphoma is a histological diagnosis made following biopsy of a lymph node or an affected organ. Treatment and prognosis are critically dependant on the histological diagnosis, which is currently defined by The World Health Organization (WHO) classification.[1] Broadly speaking, the lymphomas are subdivided into non-Hodgkin's lymphoma (NHL) and Hodgkin's disease. NHL is subdivided into high-grade and low-grade disease, and by the cell of origin either B cell or T cell.

Of all cases of non-Hodgkin's lymphoma, 85% are either follicular lymphoma (a type of low-grade disease that runs an indolent course) or diffuse large cell lymphoma (a type of high-grade disease that runs an aggressive course).

Other forms of NHL, such as mantle cell lymphoma and malt lymphomas are less common. Hodgkin's disease is subdivided into the classical-type Hodgkin's disease, which accounts for the great majority of patients with Hodgkin's disease, and nodular lymphocyte predominant Hodgkin's disease (Table 2.1).

The Ann Arbor staging system

The Ann Arbor staging system describes the extent and distribution of lymphoma (Table 2.2). This is determined by a combination of clinical assessment, bone marrow biopsy, and computed tomography (CT) scanning of the chest, abdomen, and pelvis. The suffix B is given to patients presenting with either drenching night sweats sufficient to warrant the changing of sheets or night clothes, weight loss of greater than 10% in the previous 6 months, or unexplained fevers >38 °C. Patients without B symptoms are given the suffix A. Treatment is dictated by the stage of disease at presentation. The prognosis of early (stage I and II) disease is better than advanced (stage III and IV) disease. Patients with B symptoms have a worse prognosis than those without B symptoms.

Prognostic scoring systems in lymphoma

The prognosis for patients with NHL is defined by the international prognostic index (IPI) (Table 2.3). Five-year survival for diffuse, large cell lymphoma for the four prognostic groups is low risk (75%), low intermediate risk (50%), high intermediate risk (40%), and high risk (25%). After application of the international prognostic index (IPI) for follicular lymphoma, the 10-year survival rates for the low-risk, low-intermediate risk, high-intermediate risk, and high-risk groups were 80.4%, 48.7%, 21.9%, and 0.0%, respectively.[2]

Table 2.2 The Ann Arbor staging system for lymphoma

Stage I	Disease in one lymph node area
Stage II	Disease in two or more lymph node areas on the same side of the diaphragm
Stage III	Disease in lymph node areas on both sides of the diaphragm
Stage IV	Spread of disease to extranodal tissue including bone marrow and liver
B symptoms	Weight loss >10% in 6 months, unexplained fever >38°C, drenching sweats

Table 2.3 International prognostic index for non-Hodgkin's lymphoma

Pre-treatment risk factors	Score 0	Score 1
Age in years	≤60	>60
Ann Arbor stage	I or II	III or IV
Number of extra nodal sites	One or less	>1
ECOG performance status	0 or 1	>1
Serum LDH	Normal	Raised

Risk group	Risk score
Low	0 or 1
Low intermediate	2
High intermediate	3
High	4 or 5

The Hasenclever prognostic score stratifies prognosis for patients with Hodgkin's disease. The score predicts the rate of freedom from progression of disease (see Table 2.5).

Chemotherapy treatment of classical Hodgkin's disease

First-line treatment of classical Hodgkin's disease

After histological confirmation and staging of the disease, most patients with classical Hodgkin's disease will receive treatment aimed at cure. Stage I and II disease will be treated with combination chemotherapy, e.g. three courses of ABVD (Table 2.4), followed by involved field radiotherapy. Stage III and IV disease is treated with chemotherapy (e.g. six to eight courses of ABVD). More intensive first-line therapy, such as escalated BEACOPP (with local radiotherapy for bulk disease), may improve outcome for patients with poor prognosis disease (Hasenclever score >3). The improvements in the treatment of Hodgkin's disease are based on results of previous or current randomized controlled trials. Five-year disease-free survival is approximately 90% for early stage disease and 70% for advanced stage disease. In the past, some patients were treated with high doses of radiotherapy (mantle) alone for early stage disease. In these patients relapse rate was 50% and the treatment has resulted in a high risk of breast cancer in young women.

Table 2.4 Combination chemotherapies

CHOP	Cyclophosphamide, adriamycin, vincristine, and prednisolone
ABVD	Adriamycin, bleomycin, vinblastine, and dacarbizine
ESHAP	Etoposide, methylprednisolone, cytosine arabinoside, and platinum
MBVP	Methotrexate, bleomycin, vincristine, and prednisolone

Table 2.5 Hasenclever score for Hodgkin's disease, percentage of patients and rate of freedom from progression[3]

Hasenclever score	Patients in this group (%)	Rate of freedom from progression of disease (%)
0	7	84
1	22	77
2	29	67
3	23	60
4	12	51
5 or higher	7	42

Relapsed or refractory classical Hodgkin's disease

Relapsed Hodgkin's disease is still potentially curable. Patients who have relapsed after receiving radiotherapy alone, may be cured with chemotherapy (e.g. ABVD). If the Hodgkin's disease was refractory to chemotherapy or relapsed after chemotherapy, cure can be achieved by autologous peripheral blood stem cell transplant (PBSCT) in 30–60%. Transplant-related mortality is 2–5%. Chemotherapy and radiotherapy may still be used for symptom control in patients who have incurable disease.

Nodular lymphocyte predominant Hodgkin's disease

This is much less common than classical Hodgkin's disease and is an indolent low-grade condition. Many patients never need treatment. Clinicians usually monitor these patients and treat with chemotherapy or radiotherapy only when symptoms occur; 10% transform to high-grade non-Hodgkin's lymphoma.

Chemotherapy treatment of high-grade NHL

First-line treatment of high-grade non-Hodgkin's lymphoma

Untreated, high-grade NHL has an average survival of less than one year. Stage I and II disease is treated with a combination of chemotherapy and involved field radiotherapy. Patients with stage III and IV disease are treated with chemotherapy. Following chemotherapy, radiotherapy may be given to sites of previous bulk disease. First-line anthracycline-based chemotherapy, e.g. CHOP (Table 2.4), is used to treat non-Hodgkin's lymphoma. Recently it has been shown that adding the monoclonal antibody anti-CD20 (Rituximab) to CHOP in patients over the age of 60 improves cure rates by about 15%. Studies are currently in progress to assess whether the use of anti-CD20 will improve outcomes for patients under the age of 60.

Relapsed or refractory high-grade non-Hodgkin's lymphoma

Therapy with curative intent may still be offered to patients who fail to respond to standard first-line therapy or who relapse after first-line therapy. Two-thirds of patients respond to salvage regimens such as ESHAP (Table 2.4). Of these, half can be cured with subsequent autologous PBSCT. This is not without risk and is associated with an early transplant related mortality of 2–5%.[4] The focus of treatment for patients unfit for autologous PBSCT, or who fail to respond to salvage chemotherapy, is symptom control and maintaining and improving quality of life. For a small number of young patients, allogeneic bone marrow transplant may be curative. It is, however, associated with significant morbidity and mortality.

Chemotherapy treatment of low-grade non-Hodgkin's lymphomas

Low-grade NHL mainly affects older people. These lymphomas are clinically indolent and are usually stage IV at presentation. Conventional treatment strategies are not curative but can control the disease for 5–10 years. Survival is predicted using the international prognostic index (IPI) (Table 2.3). Characteristically the course of the disease is one of recurrent remissions and relapses, and patients are usually given treatment for 6–9 months, with initial remissions lasting on average from one to two years. The duration of response to treatment falls with each successive course. Finally the disease becomes refractory to all forms of therapy. Many elderly patients die of an unrelated medical condition rather than their lymphoma, whereas younger patients are likely to die of the disease.

First-line management in low-grade non-Hodgkin's lymphoma

Very few patients with low-grade lymphoma present with localized stage I disease. Half of these can be cured with radiotherapy alone. Patients with advanced stage (II–IV) disease at diagnosis only require treatment if they have abnormal blood counts, B symptoms, or significant lymphadenopathy. Early chemotherapy does not improve survival in asymptomatic patients. Treatment is started when the patient develops symptoms—this usually takes the form of out-patient oral therapy, which has minimal side-effects (e.g. chlorambucil). Most patients respond and treatment is usually continued for 6–9 months. Some centres give more intensive treatment at presentation. There is some evidence that longer remissions are achievable with combination chemotherapy plus maintenance interferon, and at least one trial shows some survival benefit. This has to be weighed against increased side-effects from this approach.

Treatment of relapsed or refractory low-grade non-Hodgkin's lymphoma

Patients receive courses of chemotherapy when the disease recurs. Treatments include further courses of chlorambucil, fludarabine alone or in combination with an anthracycline, steroids, CHOP, antibody treatments (e.g. Rituximab and Campath), and radiotherapy. All are effective for variable periods but typically for 6–12 months. Younger patients may be offered autologous PBSCT as a form of palliative therapy at some stage during their disease. Allogeneic bone marrow transplant may be curative in a selected group of younger patients but is associated with significant risk of infection and graft versus host disease.

Palliative care in patients with lymphoma

Introduction

Symptoms associated with lymphoma may occur as a result of lymphadenopathy, bone marrow failure or the generalized effect of the malignancy. The choice of treatment depends on the clinical context in which the symptoms occur. The best form of symptom control is often active chemotherapy or radiotherapy. Further courses of intensive chemotherapy and/or radiotherapy, as previously described, should be the first approach considered in all patients with relapsed lymphoma. The patient, in consultation with the haematology/oncology team, will make this decision. The following discussion of the problems associated with lymphoma assumes that further intensive therapy has been considered but decided to be inappropriate. If there is no further active intensive therapy then the primary focus of treatment switches to symptom control. This may still include chemotherapy or radiotherapy but usually less intensive and associated with fewer side-effects than the treatments the patient may have received earlier in the course of the disease. Lymphomas frequently respond quickly to steroids. Intravenous dexamethasone 8 mg intravenously immediately followed by 4 mg four times a day can be very effective at rapidly reducing disease bulk in an emergency. Response, however, is usually short-lived unless further therapy is given to consolidate the response. Drugs, which relieve symptoms without having an anti-tumour effect, are useful either in parallel with chemotherapy or on their own. Pure symptom control may be all that can be offered in the end.

Specific problems brought about by the tumour mass

More general symptom control advice is found in Chapter 8.

Lymphadenopathy

Lymphadenopathy is common in lymphoma and produces a variety of symptoms. The symptoms depend on two factors: first, the site of the disease; and, second, the size of the disease. The main lymph node groups are situated in the mediastinum, neck, axillae, groins, and retroperitoneum.

Superior vena cava obstruction (SVCO) Superior vena caval obstruction and large airways obstruction are distressing and are a medical emergencies. Symptoms include headache and dusky discoloration and oedema of the face, chest, and arms. If the tumour compresses large airways, the patient may report shortness of breath. On examination, distended veins may be visible over the chest wall and arms. Auscultation may reveal stridor, wheeze, or reduced air entry in the chest. If SVCO is suspected in a patient with known lymphoma, intravenous dexamethasone should be started immediately. Diagnosis of SVCO may be confirmed by chest X-ray or CT scan and the patient should be considered for urgent chemotherapy and or radiotherapy.

If radiotherapy or further drug treatment is considered inappropriate, adequate analgesia and sedation should be given to prevent distress. Diamorphine and midazolam may be given subcutaneously by syringe driver at doses that provide symptom relief. Noisy breathing may be treated with hyoscine butylbromide 60–120 mg subcutaneously over 24 h by continuous infusion, and is frequently used in combination with diamorphine.

In patients presenting with the symptoms and signs of SVCO but without a known underlying malignancy, every effort should be made to obtain tissue for histological diagnosis before giving steroids or radiotherapy. This may not always be possible, and the patient's health should not be compromised by the delay.

Lymphadenopathy in the neck Lymphadenopathy in the neck obstructing the oesophagus and trachea may result in shortness of breath, stridor, wheeze, and dysphagia. In severe cases, patients are not able to swallow their own saliva, which is a very distressing symptom. Lymphadenopathy may be reduced by dexamethasone and emergency radiotherapy. The haematolologist may consider other therapies to reduce size of the lymph nodes. Intravenous vincristine 2 mg monthly or oral etoposide 50 mg once daily may be effective, even in multiply treated patients. Endobronchial stents may be considered in patients with large airway compression as a method of maintaining the patency of the airway until chemotherapy or radiotherapy can be arranged. With low-grade disease that has become refractory to chemotherapy and radiotherapy, patients may be better served with a syringe driver containing a combination of analgesia and sedation.

Lymphadenopathy in the axillae and groins The principal problems associated with axillary and inguinal lymphadenopathy are pain, swelling, and loss of limb function. Disease in the groin, pelvis, or axilla may lead to thrombosis in the great veins, which may be complicated by pulmonary emboli. Steroids and radiotherapy are usually effective in reducing the size of the nodes and reducing the compressive symptoms. Cytotoxic chemotherapy may also be considered to reduce disease bulk. Low molecular weight heparin may be considered for the prophylaxis and treatment of venous thrombo-embolism. In terminally ill patients the clinician may feel that the investigation and treatment of suspected venous thrombosis is not appropriate.

Bowel obstruction Bowel obstruction is uncommon, even in advanced disease. Patients may present with abdominal pain, distension, vomiting, and constipation. Radiotherapy to the bowel is technically difficult as the bowel may move between planning and treatment, and therefore drug therapy to reduce bulk should be used if appropriate. Surgery is rarely appropriate but should be considered for suitable patients. The medical management of bowel obstruction is outlined in Chapter 8 but a combination of an anti-emetic (such as cyclizine) with diamorphine for pain relief, administered by subcutaneous infusion, may be all that is required. Hyoscine butylbromide (60–120 mg in

24 h) with or without octreotide (300–600 µg) can be used to reduce the volume of gastric secretions, portal blood flow, and gut motility. Naso-gastric intubation should not be used routinely.

Hydronephrosis Retroperitoneal lymphadenopathy may cause ureteric obstruction and renal failure. Patients may still produce large quantities of urine despite obstructive uropathy. The obstruction can be relieved by nephrostomies. This is a short-term solution, as they are unsightly, uncomfortable, difficult to manage, and are an infection risk. After the insertion of nephrostomies, attempts need to be made either to reduce tumour bulk or insert ureteric stents. Renal failure can be managed using anti-emetics and sedatives in patients where a nephrostomy is considered inappropriate.

Bone marrow failure

Cytopenias cause tiredness, infection, and bleeding, and occur because of either reduced blood cell production or increased blood cell loss. Normal haematopoiesis is suppressed by bone marrow infiltration and chemotherapy drugs. Survival of blood cells is reduced by bleeding, splenomegaly, autoimmune haemolysis, autoimmune thrombocytopenia, and disseminated intravascular coagulation (DIC). This may result in anaemia, leucopenia, and thrombocytopenia, all of which may be severe. The management starts with correctly identifying the principal causes of the cytopenias.

Anaemia is the easiest problem to correct. First, identify the cause of the anaemia. Bleeding should be treated supportively with fluid and red cell transfusion. Attempts should be made to identify and treat the source of blood loss. Jaundice, orange discoloration of urine, and a positive direct antiglobulin test are the hallmarks of autoimmune haemolysis. This usually responds to prednisolone 1 mg/kg, orally once a day. Because of the increased risk of steroid-induced gastric bleeding and folate deficiency, patients should also receive prophylactic H_2 antagonists or proton pump inhibitors and folic acid, 5 mg daily. Bone marrow infiltration and failure is managed with supportive transfusion. The decision to transfuse an anaemic patient should not be based on the level of haemoglobin but on the patient's symptoms.

Transfusion with irradiated blood products is needed for patients with Hodgkin's disease, those who have received purine analogues (e.g. fludarabine), and following bone marrow transplant. For patients with bone marrow failure, subcutaneous erythropoietin can reduce the requirement for blood transfusion (see Chapter 10 on the management of anaemia).

As the white count drops, the risk of infection increases. With neutrophil counts of less $0.5 \times 10^9/l$, spontaneous life-threatening infection may occur. The risk is highest in patients receiving cytotoxic chemotherapy. For patients with recurrent infection, prophylactic antibiotics (ciprofloxacin 250 mg twice a day) and antifungal (fluconazole 50 mg three times a week) treatments should be considered. The drug treatment of febrile neutropenia depends on the clinical situation at the time and each case has to be judged on its own merits. Broad-spectrum oral treatments include clavulanic acid–amoxycillin combinations 375 mg three times a day or, in penicillin-sensitive patients, clarithromycin 500 mg twice a day with ciprofloxacin 500 mg twice a day. Intravenous broad-spectrum antibiotics (e.g. tazocin and gentamicin) provide the most effective treatment.

Bleeding risk is related to the degree of thrombocytopenia. Patients with platelets of greater than $50 \times 10^9/l$ are not at a significantly greater risk of bleeding than those with normal platelet counts. As the platelets fall below $50 \times 10^9/l$, the risk of bleeding increases. There should be careful consideration of the risk–benefit ratio of anticoagulants in thrombocytopenic patients and there should be a very good reason for giving warfarin or aspirin to patients with platelets of less than $50 \times 10^9/l$. Discussion with a haematologist may be helpful in making a decision. Tranexamic acid 1 g three times a day is useful in treating minor bleeding such as gum bleeding or nosebleeds. If bleeding is more severe, clotting studies should be carried out to exclude other causes such as DIC. Bleeding in patients with platelets of less than $20 \times 10^9/l$ may be treated with platelet transfusions. Platelet transfusions provide only a temporary benefit and platelets should only be given after discussion with a haematologist. Regular platelet transfusions are occasionally given to prevent bleeding but only after discussion with a haematologist. As with other areas of palliative care there are occasions where sedation is the most appropriate form of management for bleeding and cytopenic patients.

Splenomegaly Splenomegaly frequently causes pain and may contribute to pancytopenia. The pain associated with splenomegaly is often described as dragging, aching, or stitch-like pain. Generally the symptoms get worse as the spleen gets bigger. Splenectomy provides significant benefit for many patients, but carries the risk of surgery and post-operative infection. Radiotherapy to the spleen may be given. If, however, the spleen is enlarged beyond the umbilicus, the dose of radiotherapy required is generally too large for the patient to tolerate. Embolization of the splenic vessels by an interventional radiologist can reduce splenomegaly. Transiently, the pain may worsen as the spleen infarcts and patients may suffer fevers or rigors. For patients with persisting splenomegaly, analgesics and supportive blood transfusion are given to control the symptoms.

Cerebral lymphoma and spinal cord compression Primary cerebral lymphoma is a difficult disease to treat and is usually confined to the central nervous system. Often the patients are elderly and the regimens that potentially offer a cure are very intensive and cannot be tolerated by the majority. Almost all patients appear to have a good response to all initial therapies. Treatments include dexamethasone 20 mg daily for four days a month, vincristine 2 mg intravenously monthly, radiotherapy and combinations such as MBVP and high dose methotrexate. Unfortunately, disease response is short and within 12 months the symptoms often return. At this point very little is effective in terms of reducing the disease. Somnolence, confusion, and focal neurological defects are common. These patients often require a significant amount of personal care in the terminal phase of the disease. Even the most willing families will struggle at home and full nursing care is almost always required in the end.

Advanced-stage systemic lymphoma may affect the central nervous system. Diagnosis is usually confirmed by examination of the cerebrospinal fluid (CSF). Tumour cells in the cerebrospinal fluid indicate meningeal disease. A CT scan, to exclude raised intracranial pressure, is mandatory prior to lumbar puncture in patients with suspected neurological disease. Only three drugs may be given intrathecally: methotrexate 12.5 mg, cytosine arabinoside 50 mg, and hydrocortisone 100 mg. One or a combination of all three drugs is given usually weekly until clearance, and from then on monthly, often with significant symptomatic benefit.

Lymphoma may cause spinal cord compression, which is a medical emergency. Initial treatment is with dexamethasone 8 mg intravenously, followed by appropriate chemotherapy or local radiation, and dexamethasone 4 mg four times a day. An urgent MRI scan will identify the sites of cord compression.

Gastro-intestinal lymphoma and ascites Lymphoma in the gastro-intestinal tract may cause malabsorption, weight loss, and diarrhoea. The diarrhoea can be difficult to manage. Regular loperamide 2 mg with each loose stool and codeine phosphate 30 mg four times a day may help. For the uncomfortable peri-anal burning associated with the diarrhoea, topical lignocaine gel provides relief. Tense ascites can be troublesome. Diuretics (frusemide and spirinolactone) can be tried but are often of limited value. Temporary ascitic drains provide rapid symptomatic relief but are protein-losing, and often the ascites returns quickly without further chemotherapy. When the drain is in, aim to take off 1.5 l, then clamp for 4 h, then drain 1.5 l more. Continue to drain and clamp until drained to dryness. If, after removal of the drain, the site continues to ooze, an ileostomy bag can be put over the drain site.

Pleural effusions As with ascites, pleural effusions may be a recurrent troublesome problem. In the absence of chemotherapeutic response, repeated drainage may be necessary.

Cutaneous lymphoma Advanced cutaneous lymphoma is a disease that is often refractory to treatment and remissions are usually short-lived. Isolated areas may be treated with superficial radiotherapy. Diffuse disease may lead to widespread breakdown of the skin, itching, and exfoliation. Topical aqueous creams and steroids may provide some relief. Infections in the broken-down skin should be treated early with antibiotics (e.g. amoxycillin 500 mg three times a day and flucloxacillin 1 g four times a day).

Paraneoplastic problems for patients with lymphoma

Weight loss is a common problem for terminally ill patients, which can result in an upsetting change in appearance and generalized weakness. Malnourished patients have delayed wound healing and an increased susceptibility to infection. Anorexia can occur as a direct result of the tumour or may occur as a side-effect of drug therapy. Early involvement of a dietician can be helpful. Nutritional support drinks can be used to supplement the diet. Naso-gastric feeding and parenteral nutritional support is very rarely indicated in terminally ill patients. Dexamethasone and progestogens can be used to stimulate appetite.

Sweats are common in patients with lymphoma. The sweats are drenching and commonly occur at night, when it is not unusual for patients to have to change their sheets and bedclothes. This is a difficult problem to treat but steroids may be helpful.

Itch can be very distressing and patients may scratch so much their skin bleeds. Itching is particularly associated with Hodgkin's disease. Numerous treatments are available but none of these are universally successful. Treatments include Eurax cream topically, piriton 4 mg orally three times a day and cimetidine 400 mg orally daily.

More details can be found in Chapter 13.

Fevers may not always represent underlying infection. The symptom of fever is tiring for the patient. After infection has been excluded, regular paracetamol 1 g orally four times a day may be helpful.

Hypercalcaemia causes constipation, confusion, and abdominal pain. Intravenous fluids initially lower the serum calcium but this should be followed by intravenous bisphosphonate (e.g. pamidronate 90 mg) for a sustained response. The dose of pamidronate needs to be adjusted in renal failure.

Neurological paraneoplastic syndromes are rare. Patients can experience a wide variety of symptoms depending on which part of the nervous system is affected. A Guillain-Barre type pattern may occur with progressive lower motor neurone flaccid weakness and absent reflexes, starting peripherally and spreading proximally. Cerebellar syndromes often present with ataxia and dizziness. Cranial nerve palsies are less common. The diagnosis is one of exclusion. CT scan of the head needs to be performed to exclude an intracerebral mass or bleed. Lumbar puncture will exclude meningeal disease. Prognosis is very poor if patients develop a paraneoplastic neurological syndrome with average survival less than 6 months. Treatment is aimed at reducing the effects of the symptoms and the distress they cause.

Special considerations for patients who have had bone marrow transplant

Bone marrow (and stem cell) transplants can be autologous (where the patient's own bone marrow or stem cells are used) or allogeneic (where the bone marrow or stem cells come from another person).

Autologous stem cell transplantation is a technique used to allow high doses of chemotherapy to be administered. Stem cells are collected from the patient's blood or bone marrow before chemotherapy is given. Freezing preserves the stem cells. Chemotherapy is then given at high doses with the aim of destroying as much tumour as possible. These doses of treatment would permanently destroy the recipient's blood-making ability and eventually lead to death by infection or bleeding. Recovery of bone marrow and blood production is achieved by returning the frozen stem cells to the patient after the chemotherapy has been cleared from the body. 5% of patients undergoing this procedure die of infection or bleeding.

Allogeneic transplant is rarely used in the management of lymphoma. Treatment is carried out in specialist transplant centres and the patients are young. The aim of allogeneic transplant is to cure the disease by administering high doses of chemotherapy and using the donor immune system to destroy the patient's lymphoma. There is a significant risk of death from bone marrow failure, infection, and graft versus host disease (GvHD). Mortality in the first 100 days following transplant is in the region of 25%. Patients frequently require blood product support, which needs to be irradiated. Because of the high risk of fungal, viral, and bacterial infection, patients routinely receive prophylactic antimicrobial drugs. Graft versus host disease (GvHD) is a life-threatening, disabling, and extremely unpleasant complication of allogeneic bone marrow transplant. Acute GvHD occurs in the first 100 days after the transplant and characteristically causes jaundice, diarrhoea, and a widespread erythematous rash. Chronic GvHD occurs after 100 days and can affect any organ. Common patterns of chronic GvHD are: a scleroderma-type skin disorder, sore mouth, chronic alopecia, skin hyperpigmentation, and liver failure. Treatment of both acute and chronic GvHD is aimed at suppressing the immune system to prevent the graft attacking the host, and includes high-dose steroids, cyclosporin, mycophenolate, and thalidomide. The management of allogeneic bone marrow transplant patients and GvHD requires regular consultation with a bone marrow transplant specialist. This is a highly specialized area of medicine, of which few doctors have much experience and where a specialist should always be consulted.

Psychosexual problems for patients with lymphoma A quarter of patients treated for lymphoma report moderate or severe psychological distress. Many patients have to give up work and suffer financial hardship. Infertility may occur following chemotherapy and is ubiquitous following allogeneic bone marrow transplant. Impotence may occur as a result of the emotional trauma but treatable endocrine causes, such as hypothyroidism and low testosterone, should be excluded. Hair loss is common with chemotherapy. Lymphoma of the skin or face may be disfiguring. Re-integration into society may be difficult but can be helped by psychological support, cosmetic advice, and wigs. Depression is probably under-reported and anti-depressants and specialist psychiatric intervention may be helpful in selected patients.

Complications of chemotherapy and radiotherapy Common immediate symptoms related to chemotherapy include nausea, vomiting, and leucopenia. Nausea and vomiting are easily prevented by anti-emetics. Leucopenia is associated with an increased risk of life-threatening infection, which is greatest in patients with a neutrophil count less than 0.5×10^9/l. Antibiotics (ciprofloxacin 250 mg twice a day) reduce the risk of bacterial infection in neutropenic patients. Fluconazole 50 mg three times a week reduces the risk of mucosal candidiasis in neutropenic patients.

Long-term complications

Long-term toxicities are becoming increasingly important as survival following treatment for lymphoma improves. Anthracycline drugs, commonly used in the treatment of lymphoma, are associated with dose-dependent cardiac toxicity. A dose of adriamycin above 450 mg/m^2 over a lifetime may cause irreversible heart failure. If heart failure develops, ACE inhibitors may improve symptoms. Radiotherapy may cause severe mucositis leading to mouth ulcers and indigestion. Oral morphine mouthwash and proton pump inhibitors may provide relief (see Chapter 7). Following radiotherapy, the skin becomes sensitive to the sun and patients should be warned about the increased risk of sunburn. Longer term radiotherapy to the chest is associated with a risk of ischaemic heart disease, and radiotherapy to the neck is associated with an increased risk of atheroma in the carotid arteries and stroke. Both chemotherapy and radiotherapy are associated with an increased risk of second malignancy.

Second malignancies The most serious long-term complication for survivors of lymphoma is secondary malignancy. Myelodysplasia and leukaemia affects up to 5% of patients treated with combination chemotherapy and bone marrow transplants. Leukaemia following previous chemotherapy responds poorly to therapy when compared with *de novo* disease. The widespread use of mantle radiotherapy in the past for mediastinal lymphoma has left a significant number of women at high risk of developing breast cancer. The risk is greatest the younger the patient was at the time of treatment. For women who received mantle radiotherapy before the age of 20, the risk of developing breast cancer is 50% over 20 years.

Support for patients with lymphoma and their families

There are a number of sources of support for people affected by lymphoma. The general practioner, specialist nurse, and hospice services are valuable sources of support. The hospital palliative care team made up of doctors and specialist nurses can provide regular specialist medical advice, emergency treatment of symptoms, emotional support, and information about the disease. Information is also available in written form and on-line from support groups such as BACUP and the Leukaemia Research Fund. Emotional support is often given to the patient by family members who may benefit from support themselves during the time of illness or after the patient has died. Respite care can be invaluable for relatives during the patient's terminal illness.

References

1 Jaffe, E. S. *et al.* (ed.) *World Health Organization classification of tumours. Tumours of haematopoietic and lymphoid tissues.* Oxford University Press.
2 Kondo, E., Ogura, M., Kagami, Y. *et al.* (2001) Assessment of prognostic factors in follicular lymphoma patients. *Int J Hematol,* **73** (3), 363–8.
3 Hasenclever, D. and Diehl, V. (1998) A prognostic score for advanced Hodgkin's disease. International prognostic factors project on advanced Hodgkin's disease. *N Engl J Med,* **339** (21), 1506–14.
4 Mills, W., Chopra, R., McMillan, A. *et al.* (1995) BEAM chemotherapy and autologous bone marrow transplantation for patients with relapsed or refractory non-Hodgkin's lymphoma. *J Clin Oncol,* **13** (3), 588–95.

Further reading

Child, J. A., Jack, A. S., and Morgan, G. J. *The lymphoproliferative disorders.* Chapman and Hall Medical.
Hoffbrand, A. V., Lewis, S. M., and Tuddenham, E. G. D. *Postgraduate haematology* (4th edn). Butterworth Heineman.
Twycross, R., Wilcock, A., and Thorp, S. *Palliative care formulary.* Radcliffe Medical Press.

Chapter 3

Management of acute leukaemias

Santiago Pavlovsky, Pablo Desmery, and
María Cecilia Dignani

Epidemiology, diagnosis, and treatment of acute leukaemia

Acute leukaemia is a clonal neoplastic disease with proliferation of immature cells of the haematopoietic system. The leukaemic cells accumulate in the bone marrow, replacing the normal haematopoietic cells. The patient develops anaemia from the lack of red cell production and is easily fatigued and breathless. The fall in megakaryocyte and platelet production results in the patient bruising and bleeding spontaneously, or on minimal trauma—such as brushing their teeth. The failure of the myeloid system causes neutropenia with resulting infectious complications.

The acute leukaemias can be divided into lymphoblastic (ALL) and myeloblastic (AML). They represent less than 3% of all the neoplastic diseases. However, they are the leading cause of cancer death in developing countries in people under 35 years of age. Leukaemia is commoner in males. The incidence rates are similar all over the world and have not changed in the last four decades.[1]

The diagnosis of acute leukaemia is suggested by history and physical examination, and is confirmed by blood counts, and the examination of a blood film and bone marrow aspirate. In patients with a previous myelodysplastic syndrome, anaemia, leucopoenia, and/or thrombocytopenia may have appeared several months or years earlier. The use of morphology, cytochemistry, cytogenetic and molecular analysis allows differentiation into subtypes of AML or ALL. The French–American–British (FAB) group divided the AML into eight subtypes (M0–M7) and the ALL into three subtypes (L1–L3).

The World Health Organization (WHO) published a new classification of tumours of haematopoietic and lymphatic tissues in 2001[2] incorporating morphology, cytogenetics, molecular genetics, and immunological markers. Its purpose is to structure a classification that is universally applicable and prognostically relevant.

The four most important prognostic factors in both types of acute leukaemia are the age, WBC counts, cytogenetics studies at diagnosis, and time to achieve complete remission. Increasing age, high WBC counts, several abnormalities of chromosomes such as 5 or 7, trisomy 8, t(9;11) and t(9;22), and delay in achieving complete remission, conferred a worse prognosis in response rate, duration of event-free survival, and overall survival.

Acute myeloid leukaemia

The incidence of AML is 2.5/100 000 people, and increases progressively with age, reaching 15/100 000 at 75 years of age and above. The average age at diagnosis for AML is 65 years old. The incidence of AML in children is higher in the first year of life.

Since 1985, AML was subdivided according to the French–American–British (FAB) classification into eight subtypes (M0–M7) using morphological and cytochemical parameters.

The WHO classification of the AML included four major categories:

♦ AML with recurrent genetic abnormalities as t(8;21); inv(16) and t(15;17) (PML/RARα)

♦ AML with multi-lineage dysplasia mainly following a myelodysplastic syndrome (MDS) or myeloproliferative disorders

♦ AML and MDS therapy related, occurring after alkylating agent chemotherapy/radiotherapy and topoisomerase II inhibitors

♦ AML not otherwise categorized, is morphology based and reflects the other FAB classifications such as M0, M1, M2, M4, M5, M6, and M7.

The most common induction therapy is 3 days of an anthracycline (daunorubicin, mitoxantrone, or idarubicin) and 7–10 days of cytarabine. The results of this induction treatment in patients with AML aged less than 60 years was an age-dependant complete response (CR) rate of 60–80% rate. The addition of a third drug, such as thioguanine or etoposide, did not show additional benefit. A consolidation with high-dose cytarabine 12–18 g in 3–6 days with 2 days of an anthracycline, improved the disease-free survival and cure rate in patients under the age of 60 compared with low or intermediate doses of cytarabine. The use of maintenance therapy is controversial and at present only used by the German Cooperative Group.

Acute promyelocytic leukaemia (M3)

The use of ATRA in combination with an anthracycline during induction and consolidation and, in some studies, maintenance treatment with intermittent ATRA plus 6-mercaptopurine and methotrexate, has provided 75–85% of complete remission and that includes 70–80% cure. Those patients who are detected early with a molecular relapse (PML/RARα positive), still have a high rate of cure with similar induction treatment and an autologous transplantation. Other agents active in APML include arsenic trioxide, which is currently under investigation.

The use of haematopoietic growth factors (G-CSF or GM-CSF) during induction has been investigated to see if the incidence of neutropenia and fever in older patients could be reduced. However, the rate of treatment-related mortality and of complete remission showed no difference compared with control groups in several randomized studies.

Stem cell transplants

The role of haematopoietic stem cell transplant (autologous or allogeneic) in first or second complete remission is controversial and much depends on the strategy of each medical institution or clinical trial.

Allogeneic stem cell transplantation, from HLA-compatible sibling donors, may be offered to patients less than 50 years of age with standard or poor risk AML. The transplant-related mortality is increased over 35 years due to several factors including graft versus host disease (GvHD), infections, and interstitial pneumonitis, and therefore decisions about transplantation must be made on an individual basis in consultation with the patient. Only 10% of patients with AML are eligible for a sibling allogeneic transplantation.

Autologous stem cell transplantation has been increasingly used in patients under 65 with AML but there is no proven benefit in overall survival for transplant performed in first remission. Autologous transplants with marrow stored in first remission may be useful to consolidate a second remission.

Acute lymphoblastic leukaemias

The incidence rate is 1.3/100 000 people with a peak incidence at 4 years with 75% of cases occurring in children under 6 years of age. Two phenotypical groups of acute lymphoblastic leukaemias (ALL) have been described: precursor B cell and T cell lymphoblastic leukaemia, B cell ALL occurs in 80–85% and T cell ALL in about 15% of childhood ALL, and 25% adult ALL. Adverse prognostic factors include very young age (<1-year-old), and age over 10 years old, the t(9;22) and t(4;11), high white blood cell count, and late response.

A mature B cell leukaemia, FAB L3, comprises around 3% of all ALL. It is composed of medium-sized B cells with basophilic cytoplasm and numerous cytoplasmic lipid vacuoles and mitotic figures. Morphology is identical to the Burkitt lymphoma. The disease is highly aggressive but potentially curable.

Treatment

The treatment of ALL has significantly changed the prognosis, in the last three decades, in children under the age of 12 with 70–85% long-term survival. In adults the prognosis is significantly poorer with 5-year survival rates of 30–40% only. The treatment of children and young adults is similar, using four drugs for induction therapy, several intensification phases with high doses of a combination of drugs, and, finally, maintenance therapy—at present for around two to three years. In patients with a poor prognosis, mainly slow responders and those with cytogenetic abnormalities such as t(9;22), the intensification of the treatment has shown little or no improvement in survival.

The therapy of L3 ALL, similar to Burkitt-type B cell lymphoma, consists of very intensive chemotherapy of relatively short duration with 80–90% survival.

Autologous stem cell transplantation used early in poor-risk patients or after relapse has shown no statistically difference over conventional chemotherapy.

Allogeneic stem cell transplantation, using HLA-compatible donors (related or unrelated) is used in younger patients as consolidation of a first complete remission (in adults) in poor prognosis or in early relapse (<18 months). In these cases, randomized and historical control studies have shown advantage over conventional therapy.

Who should receive palliative care rather than intensive chemotherapy?

ALL

Most patients with ALL are children and young adults. In view of the recent progress in managing the disease, all should be offered intensive chemotherapy and many children will be cured.

Palliative care rather than intensive chemotherapy may be the most appropriate option for those patients with co-existing serious disease, those with refractory disease after intensive treatment, or for older patients. There can be no absolute age threshold and everyone must be treated individually—the complication rate is higher above the age of 65 years. Each patient must be fully informed of the possible mortality and certain morbidity of intensive therapy.

AML

In AML, half of the patients are over the age of 65 at diagnosis and no study has demonstrated that chemotherapy increases the overall survival compared with palliative care.[3] Most of these patients should not be treated with

Table 3.1 Which patients with acute leukemia would be candidates for palliative care?

- Patients with AML and ALL over 65 years old.
- Patients with secondary AML following MDS or solid tumors over the age of 55.
- Patients with AML refractory to induction chemotherapy.
- Patients with severe comorbid disease (e.g. cardiac, renal or respiratory failure disseminated or an unresolved fungal disease).

AML: acute myeloid leukemia.

ALL: acute lymphoblastic leukemia.

MDS: myeloid displasic syndrome.

chemotherapy, as it may actually shorten their survival time and not give them the best quality of life. The length of time spent in hospital, the number of red blood cells and platelet transfusions, as well as courses of antibiotics and anti-fungal therapy, are much higher in those receiving induction chemotherapy. Also, patients under the age of 65 who have AML secondary to a myelodys-plastic syndrome or a solid tumour have very poor prognosis, and palliative care is a valid option if this is what the patient wants. In addition, patients who become refractory to first-line induction therapy or relapse early, or who develop systemic complications such as renal, respiratory, cardiac failure, or disseminated fungal infections, may have a better quality of life if they opt for palliative care only and forego disease-altering therapy (Table 3.1).

Management of clinical problems

Introduction

At the time of diagnosis of leukaemia, most patients show signs and symptoms that result from a decreased normal marrow function or infiltration by leukaemic blasts. During the course of treatment, most symptoms are related to the toxicity of the chemotherapeutic regimens and especially neutropenia-related infection and bleeding.

The clinical management of patients with leukaemia is complex, and it is outlined below.

Management of infectious complications

Infectious complications are important causes of morbidity and mortality among patients with leukaemia. These infections are usually severe and require early aggressive management, including rapid administration of broad-spectrum parenteral antibiotics. The primary goal of this treatment is to avoid infection-related mortality in a patient who will be cured of their malignancy. In these circumstances all necessary investigations, invasive procedures, and prolonged therapies should be employed.

Patients receiving palliative care

Aggressive management of infection may not be the best option for those patients when the prognosis is limited and the goal of therapy is maintaining or improving the patient's quality of life. The aims of treating infectious complications are to reduce symptoms (minimizing the number of invasive procedures) and enable the patient to be at home as much as possible. Further discussion of the issues related to treating infections will be found in Chapters 6, 8, and 15.

Bacterial infections in patients receiving palliative care

During the last decade, there have been several advances in the management of patients with neutropenia ($<0.5 \times 10^9$) and fever that have increased the survival of patients having intensive chemotherapy. It is stressed to patients, undergoing such treatment, that they must notify the hospital if they have a fever or rigors.

Several antibiotic regimens are both practical and adequate for the management of patients with neutropenia and fever in the out-patient setting. Most of these cover Gram-positive and Gram-negative bacteria.[4] The antibiotic prescribed should take into account local microbiological prevalences and sensitivity patterns.

A useful oral treatment is the combination of Amoxicillin-clavulanate (1 g bid) or clindamycin (300 mg qid) plus ciprofloxacin (750 mg bid). Similarly, examples of ambulatory parenteral regimens include: Ceftriaxone (1 g bid or 2 g/day) plus gentamicin (once daily dose 5 mg/kg) or amikacin (once daily dose of 15 mg/kg), and cefepime (2 g bid) with or without teicoplanin (8–10 mg/kg/day) or vancomycin (1 g bid). In patients with impaired renal function, the dosing interval of some antibiotics is increased and, therefore, these antibiotics (usually given at least three times a day) become suitable for use in the out-patient setting. One example is meropenem. This antibiotic should be given twice (1 g) a day in patients who have a creatinine clearance <50 ml/min. Alternatively, patients may receive parenteral antibiotics as an in-patient for a few days and then be switched to the oral route to enable them to be discharged home.

Fungal infections

The most common fungal infections that develop in patients with leukaemia include superficial candidiasis (oral and/or oesophageal) and invasive fungal infections caused by yeasts (*Candida* spp., *Trichosporon* spp.) or moulds (mainly *Aspergillus* spp. and *Fusarium* spp.).

Oral candidiasis can easily be diagnosed clinically. The definitive diagnosis of oesophageal candidiasis requires a biopsy, but in these patients it is acceptable to start empirical treatment when the diagnosis is suspected on clinical grounds. Biopsy is indicated if there is no response to this.

Superficial candidiasis can be treated with oral antifungal agents such as fluconazole (100–200 mg/day) or itraconazole (200–400 mg/day). Fluconazole (capsules or solution) is better absorbed and tolerated than itraconazole (capsules or solution) but itraconazole solution may be effective in cases of oral candidiasis that has not responded to fluconazole. Most species of *Candida* respond to these two oral antifungal agents, except for *Candid krusei*. In this case, parenteral antifungal agents (amphotericin B or any of its lipid formulations or newer agents such as caspofungin) may be used (see below). Another new agent, voriconazole, given orally or intravenously, can be active against *Candida krusei*.

Invasive candidiasis (acute or chronic disseminated candidiasis) may be treated with the oral antifungal fluconazole at high doses (400–800 mg/day), except for infections caused by *Candida krusei*. Conventional amphotericin B (0.6–1 mg/kg/day) can only be used in the in-patient setting as it has significant toxicity (renal and infusion-related). Lipid formulations of amphotericin B include liposomal amphotericin B (Ambisome), amphotericin B lipid complex (ABLC), and amphotericin B colloidal dispersion (ABCD). All these compounds are less toxic than conventional amphotericin B, however, the parenteral compounds that are suitable for out-patient treatment are liposomal amphotericin B (1–3 mg/kg/day) and potentially the new agent Caspofungin (50 mg/day).

Other invasive fungal infections are difficult both to diagnose and to treat, especially in palliative care patients. In these patients we suggest the use of non-aggressive methods for diagnosis. An accurate diagnosis of fungal pneumonia (such as *Aspergillus* spp. or *Fusarium* spp.) can be made by CT scan (positive for nodules, cavities, or halo sign), sputum culture, and clinically (no response to broad-spectrum antibiotics). The drugs of choice for the treatment of most fungal infections include all formulations of amphotericin B and itraconazole, except for infections caused by *Pseudoallescheria boydii*. In this infection, fluconazole is the drug of choice. Unless its intravenous formulation is available, itraconazole (capsules or solution) is usually used in patients in whom the infection is under control after induction treatment with any amphotericin B.[5]

The duration of treatment for invasive fungal infections varies. It should not be discontinued until there has been complete resolution both of the infection and the immunosuppression. Palliative care patients may never be cured of such infections, as they remain immunosuppressed. Antifungal treatment may therefore need to be continued indefinitely to avoid reactivation of the infection.

Viral infections

Herpes simplex (HSV) and *Varicella zoster* (VZV) are the viruses that most commonly affect patients with leukaemia. Fortunately, there are oral treatments available for both of these infections.

The majority of HSV infections are localized in the oral or nasal cavity, and may mimic chemotherapy related mucositis. In a few patients these localized infections can disseminate causing organ damage such as pneumonitis and hepatitis.

VZV infections can manifest as chickenpox or herpes zoster. *Herpes zoster* infections may be localized to a dermatome or disseminate in skin, or systemically in the central nervous system or organs such as the liver and lungs.

Oral treatments can be used for all these infections when they are confined to the skin. These treatments include acyclovir, valacyclovir, and famcyclovir. The last two drugs have a longer half-life and are better absorbed than acyclovir. The highest dosages of these antiviral agents are used for the treatment of any VZV or a disseminated HSV infection, while lower dosages can be used for localized HSV infections.

Patients who have organ damage, or who are severely affected, may be treated by intravenous therapy initially and be switched to oral treatment once the infection is under control.

Antiviral treatment should be continued until complete resolution of the infection; this is usually longer than in immunocompetent patients.

Prophylaxis

Patients with leukaemia receiving palliative care should be advised about simple infection-control measures: these mainly concern the prevention of exposure to pathogens. They should only be applied if they *do not impair* the patient's quality of life.

- *Mouth care*: antisepsis of the oral cavity is recommended for these patients, especially those who develop chemotherapy or neutropenia-related mucositis. (See Chapter 7 for more details.)

- *Hand washing*: this is the most important measure for preventing infection and it should be carried out after using the toilet, before eating, before cooking, and after touching pets.

- *Environment*: patients with leukaemia can reduce their exposure to foodborne pathogens by eating well-cooked food. Avoiding dusty areas, leaking water, and avoiding the ingestion of black pepper can reduce exposure to fungi. Parasite infection can be avoided by using gloves during gardening, being hygienic in the bathroom, and drinking potable water (ice included).

- *Pets*: these are a source of pleasure and support but can also harbour bacterial and fungal infections. Patients with leukaemia should avoid contact with their pet's secretions and excrement. They should also avoid contact with animals that are unwell.

- *Households*: the family and other members of a patient's household can transmit infections to the patient. Households can be immunized against influenza. In some countries, but not in the UK, households may also be immunized against VZV, measles, and hepatitis A. Sexual partners should also be vaccinated against hepatitis B.

- *Vaccines*: leukaemia patients who are receiving palliative care may not benefit from immunization because of their severe immunosuppression. There are three important recommendations that do apply to these patients: they should avoid contact with children who have been recently vaccinated against polio with the oral vaccine (because the polio virus can be excreted in the faeces in high concentration); they should avoid contact with children who are developing a rash related to the VZV vaccine (these lesions harbour the virus); and they should avoid injection with, or ingestion of, live vaccines (oral polio, MMR, VZV, BCG, yellow fever).

- *Post-exposure prophylaxis*: leukaemia patients should report to their physician any accidental exposure to contacts who subsequently developed an infectious disease. In some situations, these patients may benefit from post-exposure prophylaxis.

Pulmonary complications

The development of pulmonary infiltrates is a common complication after chemotherapy for AML. Recent studies have shown that in neutropenic patients who remain febrile after 48 h of antibiotic treatment, a high resolution CT scan will indicate pneumonia in 60% of cases. After these results are combined with cultures obtained by bronchoalveolar lavage (BAL), there is 87% sensitivity and 57% specificity for the diagnosis of pneumonia.[6]

One practical approach for abnormal chest X-rays is to divide them further into those with diffuse and those with focal infiltrates. Diffuse infiltrates are often due to pulmonary oedema, for which the major risk factor is old age. A trial of frusemide should be given when there is no other diagnosis. Infectious pneumonia is the commonest diagnosis when there is focal infiltration.

BAL is the most useful diagnostic procedure and it has the lowest complication rate; it has become the cornerstone for the diagnosis of pulmonary infiltrates during thrombocytopenia. Other alternatives, such as CT scan-guided needle aspiration and open-lung biopsy, are used only in selected patients.

BAL should be used early in the course of the disease, a number of different studies have clearly demonstrated that the chances of survival are related to the positive diagnosis of lung infection. In fact, the chance of leaving hospital alive increased from 20 to 60% due to this diagnosis being made.

Alveolar haemorrhage is a syndrome related to advanced disease, thrombocytopenia, and renal dysfunction. There is no good evidence for the efficacy of any treatment but steroids (>3 mg/kg/day of prednisone) and frequent platelet transfusions are those most frequently used.

Respiratory support

The very poor prognosis of patients with leukaemia who receive invasive mechanical ventilation has been consistently shown in observational studies over more than three decades. This has encouraged the development of alternative methods of treating respiratory failure.

At the end of the 1990s, prospective randomized trials generated strong evidence that non-invasive ventilation (NIV) should be the first treatment option in neutropenic or immunocompromised patients who develop respiratory failure. In a well-designed trial by Hilbert et al.[7] NIV was compared to the standard approach (oxygen and endotracheal intubation). The results were impressive, they showed a reduction in the need of endotracheal intubation from 77% in the standard approach to 46% with NIV and, even more important, hospital mortality was reduced from 80 to 50%. The number of patients that needed to be treated in order to prevent one hospital death was 3.3. Intermittent NIV reduced dyspnoea and was associated with recovery in patients with advanced disease, relapsed disease, and even in those who refused to be placed on invasive mechanical ventilation. The benefits of NIV were also seen in the paediatric population.

Gastro-intestinal complications

Nausea and vomiting

More information will be found in Chapters 6 and 8.

The emesis induced with the standard induction regimen—cytarabine ($<$1g/m^2) and anthracyline drugs (doxorubicin, mitoxantrone or idarubicin)—can be controlled with metoclopramide and serotonin receptor antagonists (e.g. ondansetron 8 mg/day IV) plus dexamethasone (10–20 mg). After relapse, chemotherapy toxicity usually rises because of the introduction of treatments that include high-dose cytarabine (>1 g/m^2 × 6–8 doses), cyclophosphamide or methotrexate. Nausea and vomiting can be controlled completely in 50–70% of people with the combination of the drugs mentioned above.

Diarrhoea and abdominal pain

Diarrhoea and abdominal pain may be the presenting symptoms of neutropenic enterocolitis, which is an acute inflammatory disease that may involve caecum, colon, and the terminal part of the ileum. The neutropenia, infection, and drug-induced alteration of bowel mucosa surface may play a role in the aetiology of this condition. Food intake is commonly significantly limited, leading to the use of total parental nutrition. Opioids may be required to control the severe abdominal pain that occurs. The use of ultrasonography has recently been described for stratifying patients with neutropenic enterocolitis. Those patients who are symptomatic, and who have bowel wall thickening detected on ultrasonography, have a higher mortality rate than patients with symptoms but no thickening of the bowel wall. In addition, patients with a bowel wall thickness of more than 10 mm require total parenteral nutrition and antibiotics to rest the bowel because their prognosis is poor.[8]

Renal dysfunction

This is common in the treatment of acute leukaemia and is often multifactorial. Recognition of the risk and the prevention of tumour lysis syndrome are essential.

Adequate fluid replacement and 10 mg/kg of allopurinol are crucial to avoid renal damage related to tumour lysis syndrome at the beginning of treatment of acute leukaemia.

During neutropenia, renal toxicity and sepsis-induced renal failure are relatively common; no specific therapy is indicated except for the adjustment of toxic drugs such as amphotericin B and aminoglycosides. The use of renal doses of dopamine (less than 5 mg/kg/min) did not benefit patients.

Nutritional support

Patients with acute leukaemia develop malnutrition due to chemotherapy related gastro-intestinal toxicity, especially if they develop neutropenic enterocolitis or viral infections such as those caused by *Herpes simplex*. Enteral nutrition is the preferred route for feeding patients with leukaemia when the gastro-intestinal tract is functional. It can be accomplished in the vast majority of patients by using supplementation between meals. Thrombocytopenia limits the use of naso-gastric feeding tubes, although after platelet transfusion the risk of bleeding is low. Total parenteral nutrition is restricted to those patients with enterocolitis during an episode of neutropenia, when the gastro-intestinal tract must rest, or those unable to tolerate enteral supplements. If the patient is of good nutritional status, total parenteral nutrition offers little advantage over a short period of relative starvation, but if the patient is already malnourished, total parental nutrition is necessary.

Haemorrhage related to thrombocytopenia

Transfusion thresholds are related to each patient's condition and haemoglobin levels around 8 g/dl are well tolerated in the absence of coronary heart disease or hypoxemia.

Haemorrhage is a common problem in the advanced stages of acute leukaemia. Patients with platelet counts under $5–10 \times 10^5/l$, who tend to bleed, may benefit from prophylactic platelet transfusions. Patients with platelet counts less than $20 \times 10^5/l$, should receive platelet transfusions only in case of fever and/or bleeding. A proportion of patients become refractory to platelet transfusions and require HLA-matched products.

There is further discussion of about the end of life in patients with leukaemia, in Chapters 14 and 15.

There is little evidence concerning the last days of patients with haematological malignancies, and most of the data that is available has been obtained from studies that were mainly concerned with patients with solid tumours.[9]

One of the few studies that is concerned with this group included 81 patients, 75% of whom had AML/ALL, lymphomas, or haematological diseases. The most frequent clinical complaint causing admission was dyspnoea, which occurred in 44% of the patients studied. Breathlessness was caused by heart failure, pulmonary infection, hyperleucocytosis, or pulmonary involvement by the disease. In addition, 40% of patients suffered from fever; 27% were admitted because of pain—most of the patients complained of abdominal pain; 20% of patients had haemorrhage—most frequently from the nose, oral cavity, rectum, retina, or central nervous system.[10]

Table 3.2 Prevalence of common symptoms in dying cancer patients

General cancer patients	(%)	Patients with haematologic malignancies	(%)
Pain	84	Dyspnea	44
Easy fatigue	69	Fever	40
Weakness	66	Pain	27
Anorexia	66	Central nervous system disturbance	25
Lack of energy	61	Haemorrhages	20
Dry mouth	57		
Constipation	52		

Table 3.3 Difference between patients with leukemia and other cancers at the end of life

	Leukemia patients	Other cancer patients
Use of permanent IV catheter	>80%	<50%
Location for the last days	Hospital	Home
Transfusion requirement	High	Low
Predominant symptoms	Dyspnea, pain and fever	Pain and gastro-intestinal complaints
Infection occurrence	Very common	Rare
Use of terminal sedation	High	20–30%

There are significant differences between the last days of patients with leukaemia and other neoplastic diseases. Table 3.2 compares the symptoms and Table 3.3 the differences in medical care of these two patient populations. Patients with leukaemia and palliative-care needs often require the facilities of a hospital because of the requirement for transfusion and antibiotic treatment. Symptom control may lead to the administration of terminal sedation and local facilities dictate whether this can be given, in a timely way, at home (Table 3.2).

Towards the end of life, half of the patients will receive palliative chemotherapy. This may be an effective mode of symptom control in haematological patients who remain chemosensitive.

References

1 Scheinberg, D. A., Maslak, P., and Weiss, M. (2001). Acute leukaemia. In *Cancer principles & practice of oncology*, (6th edn) (ed., V. T. De Vita, S. Hellman, and S. A. Rosenberg), pp. 2404–33. Lippincott-Williams & Wilkins.

2 Jaffe, E. S., Harris, N. L., Stein, H. *et al.* (2001). *World Health Organization classification of tumours of haemopoietic and lymphoid tissues.* IARC Press, Lyon.

3 Pulsoni, A., Pagano, L., Tosti, M. E. *et al.* (2000). Retrospective survival analysis of elderly patients with acute myeloid leukaemia (AML) treated with aggressive or non aggressive therapy. *Blood,* **96**, 503a.

4 Hughes, W., Armstrong, D., Bodey, G. *et al.* (2002). Guidelines for the use of antimicrobial agents in neutropenic patients with cancer. *Clin Infect Dis,* **34**, 730–51.

5 Stevens, D., Kan, V. L., Judson, M. A. *et al.* (2000). Practice guidelines for diseases caused by *Aspergillus. Clin Infect Dis,* **30**, 696–709.

6 Heussel, C. P., Kauczor, H. U., Heussel, G. E. *et al.* (1999). Pneumonia in febrile neutropenic patients and in bone marrow and blood stem-cell transplant recipients: use of high-resolution computed tomography. *J Clin Oncol,* **17**, 796–805.

7 Hilbert, G., Gruson, D., Vargas, F. *et al.* (2001). Non-invasive ventilation in immunosuppressed patients with pulmonary infiltrates, fever and acute respiratory failure. *N Eng J Med*, **344**, 481–7.

8 Cartoni, C., Dragoni, F., Micozzi, A. *et al.* (2001). Neutropenic enterocolitis in patients with acute leukaemia: prognostic significance of bowel wall thickening detected by ultrasonography. *J Clin Oncol*, **19**, 756–61.

9 Walsh, D., Donnelly, S., and Rybicki, L. (2000). The symptoms of advanced cancer: relationship to age, gender and performance status in 1000 patients. *Supportive Care Cancer*, **8**, 175–9.

10 Middlewood, S., Gardner, G., and Gardner, A. (2001). Dying in hospital: medical failure or natural outcome? *J Pain Symptom Manage*, **22**, 1035–41.

Chapter 4

Myelodysplastic syndromes

Ghulam Mufti and Kavita Raj

Introduction

The earliest reports of what is now termed myelodysplastic syndromes (MDS) date back to 1913. These were cases of anaemia that were refractory to haematinics. The blood films showed variations in red cell size and the bone marrows were discrepantly hypercellular. On follow-up the patients succumbed to progressive anaemia, infections, and haemorrhage or progressed to acute leukaemia.

In 1973 Saarni and Linman reviewed 'pre-leukaemic' anaemia and proposed that these were primarily a marrow disorder distinct from acute leukaemia, characterized by progressive peripheral cytopenias, marrow hypercellularity, disordered precursor maturation, and eventual progression to acute myeloid leukaemia.

Further refinement in diagnosis came from the French–American–British (FAB) co-operative group, which in 1976 categorized 'dysmyelopoietic syndrome' into two broad categories: refractory anaemia with excess blasts; and chronic myelomonocytic leukaemia. The group also identified a range of conditions associated with bone marrow hypercellularity, which could be mistaken for acute myeloid leukaemia.

In time it became apparent that the previous two categories did not sufficiently define features for progression to acute myeloblastic leukaemia (AML). It was also evident that this was a broad spectrum of disorders, which could be differentiated into categories based on different morphologic features, with each predicting a different risk of blastic transformation. In 1982 the term 'myelodysplastic syndromes' was used by the FAB co-operative group to encompass this group of disorders.[1] The group defined five subcategories, namely: refractory anaemia (RA), refractory anaemia with ringed sideroblasts (RARS), refractory anaemia with excess blasts (RAEB), refractory anaemia with excess blasts in transformation (RAEB-t), and chronic myelomonocytic leukaemia.

Because of their recent definition, varying nomenclature, and difficulties in making a diagnosis, the exact incidence of the myelodysplastic syndromes is not known. In North America, the Surveillance Epidemiology and End Results (SEER) Program of the National Cancer Institute does not require registration of MDS, leading to lack of reliable data. Data by Linman and Bagby from 1978 approximated 1500 new cases per year in the USA, but this is probably an underestimate as only cases with less than 5% blasts were included.

Swedish registries are fraught with further problems with MDS being registered under five different categories. However, a recent study estimated the incidence of MDS to be 3.6/100 000.

The Leukaemia Research Foundation (UK) in the 1980s estimated the incidence of MDS to be 3.6/100 000. However, there were four-fold variations in reported incidence from different counties, with centres that had a specialist interest recording the highest incidence. Bournemouth had an incidence of 12.6/100 000 and Somerset a rate of 9.3/100 000.

The age at diagnosis was older than 55 years in 90% of cases (median 69 years) with a male-to-female ratio of 1.4. The incidence increased with age to 34/100 000 in males and 17/100 000 in females in those between 75 and 79 years.

Aetiology

A wide variety of exposures have been linked with increased risk of MDS; however, in the majority of cases the influence of environmental factors remain unexplained.

Exposure to ionizing radiation has been implicated in MDS. Japanese atomic bomb survivors had an increased incidence of MDS in the high-dose exposure group. Patients with non-Hodgkin's lymphoma, breast cancer, uterine cervix cancer, uterine corpus cancer, and Ewing's sarcoma have a two- to three-fold excess risk of secondary AML, which is attributed to treatment with radiotherapy.

Chemotherapy has also been linked to subsequent development of AML and MDS. Treatment with alkylating agents, particularly melphalan, may be followed five to seven years later by MDS and therapy related AML (tAML). This risk is related to the cumulative dose of the drug. There is often a pre-leukaemic phase, trilineage dysplasia, and complex cytogenetic abnormalities involving partial deletions of chromosomes 5 and 7 are detected in over 90% of such patients.

Topoisomerase II inhibitors, especially epipodophyllotoxins, are also linked to tAML. A pre-leukaemic phase is often absent and the latency is shorter (median 2 years). Balanced translocations and or deletions involving 11q23 site of the MLL gene are often detected.

Methotrexate in combination with mitoxantrone or mitomycin C for breast cancer is associated with a 10-fold increase in risk of MDS/tAML.[2] Platinum-based chemotherapy for ovarian cancer; high-dose chemotherapy, and autologous stem cell transplantation—especially with total body irradiation or VP16 conditioning—have also been implicated in the development of future MDS/tAML.[3]

Benzene, the best-known chemical leukaemogen, is strongly associated with AML and aplastic anaemia; there is evidence to suggest that the development of MDS is also linked to exposure to it. Other chemicals, such as tetrachloro-bibenzo-p dioxin and 1,3 butadiene,[4] may also cause AML. Various pesticides, fertilizers, diesel fuel, and exhaust, alcohol, smoking, and hairdyes are suspect; viruses may also be implicated.[5]

Pathogenesis of MDS

MDS arises through the stepwise acquisition of genomic 'hits' within a multi-potent haemopoietic stem cell. Haematological abnormalities, such as peripheral blood cytopenias, are secondary to excessive apoptosis with resultant ineffective haemopoiesis.[6] Whilst the exact mechanisms underlying leukaemic transforma-tion remain unclear, various molecular targets are implicated in its evolution. Activating mutations of the RAS oncogene, which lead to unregulated cellular proliferation, and inhibition of differentiation are frequently present and are particularly common in CMML (in up to 40% of cases). NRAS mutations, involving positions 12 and 13, are particularly frequent and are associated with an increased risk of leukaemic transformation and poor prognosis. Fms encodes for the macrophage colony stimulating factor receptor and its mutations are found in 5–15% of MDS cases. Again, it is more common in CMML and confers a worse prognosis. Molecular lesions leading to aberrant expression of c-myc, c-myb, c-mos, c-kit, c-able, c-mpl, FLT3, and WT1 have all been reported. Abnormal gene methylation with silencing of genes such as $P15^{INK4b}$ has also been demonstrated in MDS. $P15^{INK4b}$ methylation is associated with a poor prognosis due to leukaemic transformation. Whilst the exact role of each of these mutations and their interplay with each other remains unclear, the end result is a dysregulated cell with abnormal differentiation and proliferation. They are therefore potential targets for therapeutic manipulation.

Alteration in gene function in MDS

Mutations of various genes are thought to mediate the pathogenesis and progression of MDS. Of these the common ones are RAS, FMS, Internal-Tandem duplication (ITD) of FLT3, and p53 genes. Hypermethylation leading to silencing of the p15INK 4b gene is also particularly common in MDS.

The RAS oncogene that encodes for RAS proteins is involved in the control of cellular proliferation, differentiation, and cell death. The proteins bind guanine nucleotides and their function is controlled by cycling between the guanosine triphosphate (GTP)-bound (active) and guanosine diphosphate (GDP)-bound (inactive) forms. Mutant RAS proteins retain the active GTP-bound form and are constitutively activated.

In MDS, NRAS mutations have been detected in 10–40% of cases. They are associated with a higher risk of transformation to AML and shorter survival. The presence of additional abnormal karyotypes increases the likelihood of transformation.

The FLT3 gene is mutated (internal tandem duplication) in 10% of cases with MDS. The gene encodes a class III receptor tyrosine kinase that plays a role in stem cell differentiation. Mutation of the gene causes activation of the product. They are associated with progression to AML and poor prognosis.

p53 gene mutations are common in MDS, being present with a frequency of 5–25% and higher in cases of therapy related MDS. The gene normally regulates cell cycle by encoding G1 and G2 checkpoint protein products that monitor integrity of genome; they arrest the cell cycle in response to DNA damage.

Loss of the wild-type allele is observed in both early and late MDS, and is associated with a rapid progression to AML particularly poor outcome. 17p, -5/del (5q), -7/del (7q) suggest pathogenic exposure to carcinogens.

P15INK4b gene is a cell cycle regulator that regulates the transition from G0 to G1 in the cell cycle. Hypermethylation of the promoter region of the gene leads to its silencing. This phenomenon is seen in upto 80% of cases with advanced MDS. The silencing of the gene can be reversed by the use of demethylating agents such as 5 azacytidine.

Cytogenetic abnormalities in MDS

Chromosomal abnormalities are detected at diagnosis in 40–70% of patients with primary MDS but in 95% of patients with therapy related MDS. The frequency of these abnormalities increases with the severity of the disease and the risk of leukaemic transformation: 15–20% of cases with RA and RARS have abnormal cytogenetics, compared to 75% of RAEB and RAEB-t cases.

Generally, the recurring abnormalities found in MDS (Table 4.1) are unbalanced with chromosomal loss and deletions, as well as unbalanced translocations commonly seen. A few cytogenetic abnormalities have been specifically associated with morphologically and clinically distinct subsets of MDS such as the 5q-syndrome, the 17p-syndrome, and the isodicentric X chromosome associated with RARS, which has a high likelihood of transformation to AML.

Table 4.1 Recurrent chromosomal abnormalities in myelodysplastic syndrome

Chromosomal loss or gain	Translocations	Deletions	Others
−5	t(1;3)(p36;q21)	5(q13q33)	inv(3)(q21;q26)
−7	t(1;7)(p11;p11)	7(q22q34)	i(17q)
−17	t(5;7)(p11;p11)	11(q14q22)	
−Y	t(2;11)(p21;q23)	12(p11p13)	
+8	t(6;9)(p23;q34)	13(q14)	
+21	t(11;21)(q24;q11)	20(q11q13)	

Monosomy 5/del (5q)

Del (5q) as an isolated anomaly may give rise to the 5q minus syndrome, characterized by female preponderance, macrocytosis, trilineage dysplasia, modest leucopenia, normal to high platelet counts, and hypolobulated micromegakaryocytes. BM blasts are usually less than 5%, although cases of RAEB and RAEB-t that fulfil the morphological criteria for 5q minus syndrome have also been described.

Interstitial deletions of the long arm of chromosome 5, del (5q), or complete chromosomal loss, is a frequent finding in MDS, MDS-AML (AML secondary to MDS) and treatment-related disease. The size of deletion on 5q varies and spans a large portion of DNA between q11 and q35. The critical region deleted in the 5q minus syndrome (5q32) is telomeric to (5q31) that is associated with MDS-AML. Several genes involved in cellular proliferation and differentiation have been mapped to the minimal deleted region at 5q31 but the identity of the target gene involved in MDS pathogenesis remains elusive. Additional cytogenetic abnormalities are frequent, most commonly involving chromosome 7.

Prognostic significance of the chromosome 5 deletions in MDS varies. In therapy related disease and in advanced MDS, del (5q)/-5 generally implies rapid leukaemic progression and poor outcome. The 5q minus syndrome however, carries a lower risk of leukaemic transformation and a favourable prognosis.

17p Deletions

17p aberrations almost invariably lead to deletions of the p53 tumour-suppresser gene located at 17p13 and are frequently accompanied by inactivating mutations of the remaining p53 allele. Clinically they are characterized by specific dysgranulopoiesis combined with pseudo-Pelger-Huet nuclear hypolobulation and vacuolated cytoplasm.

Patients typically have advanced or therapy related disease, harbour additional complex cytogenetic abnormalities, often involving chromosomes 5 and/or 7, and are at an increased risk of leukaemic transformation. They respond poorly to chemotherapy and overall survival is short.

3q Abnormalities

Breakpoints at 3q21 and 3q26 (site of the transcriptional activator MDS/EVI1) occur in MDS-AML. These patients often have prior mutagenic exposure and may have additional chromosomal aberrations, often involving chromosomes 5 and 7. The marrow shows trilineage dysplasia with micromegakaryocytic hyperplasia and the platelet count is often normal or increased. Most patients have progressive disease and respond poorly to chemotherapy.

Monosomy 7/del (7q)

These anomalies are frequently observed in MDS and AML, especially in disease arising from inherited pre-leukaemic disorders, familial disease, or following mutagenic exposure. The cytogenetic break points are variable and range from 7q11–q22 proximally to 7q31–q36 distally. There are several common deleted segments at 7q22, 7q32–q33, and 7q35–q36, with several potential candidate tumour-suppressor genes at these sites.

In MDS, it carries a poor prognosis with associations of increased susceptibility to infections, rapid disease progression, poor response to chemotherapy, and decreased survival.

Classification of MDS

The FAB classification

Described by the 1982 French–American–British morphology co-operative group based on peripheral blood and bone marrow morphology. It provided a framework for the identification of MDS patients and a common language for clinical trials (see Table 4.2).

The classification does not take into account secondary or therapy related MDS, novel subgroups with distinct cytogenetic and morphologic features, nor does it incorporate the overlap syndromes between aplastic anaemia, myeloproliferative disorders, and myelodysplastic syndrome.

The WHO classification of MDS

The World Health Organization guidelines for the classification of malignant haematological disorders (1999) recognized six categories of MDS[7] (see Table 4.3).

Table 4.2 French–American–British (FAB) classification of myelodysplastic syndrome

FAB subgroup	Peripheral blood criteria	Bone marrow criteria
Refractory anaemia (RA)	Blasts <1%, monocytes <1 × 10⁹/l and	Blasts <5%, ringed sideroblasts <15% of erythroblasts
Refractory anaemia with ringed sideroblasts (RARS)	Blasts <1%, monocytes <1 × 10⁹/l and	Blasts <5%, ringed sideroblasts >15% of erythroblasts
Refractory anaemia with excess blasts (RAEB)	Blasts >1%, <5%, monocytes <1 × 10⁹/l and/or	Blasts 5–19%
Refractory anaemia with excess blasts in transformation (RAEB-t)	Blasts > 5% or auer rods or	Blasts 20–29% or auer rods
Chronic myelomonocytic leukaemia	Blasts <5%, monocytes >1 × 10⁹/l	Blasts up to 20%, promonocytes/monocytes often increased

Table 4.3 Who classification of adult myelodysplastic syndrome

Refractory anaemia: <5% blasts, unilineage dysplasia

Refractory anaemia with ringed sideroblasts (RARS):
  <5% blasts
  15% ringed sideroblasts
  unilineage dysplasia

Refractory cytopenia with multilineage dysplasia (RCMD):
  <5% blasts
  2/3 lineage dysplasia

Refractory anaemia with excess blasts (RAEB):
  5–20% blasts
  myelodysplasia

MDS unclassified:
  Insufficient/unsuitable material for analysis
  Failure to categorise in the above categories

5q-syndrome

1. Auer rods within the myeloid precursors does not influence allocation to a particular MDS subtype.
2. CMML will be incorporated within the myeloproliferative disorders.
3. RAEB-t is eliminated; AML is classified as clonal disease with >20% blasts.

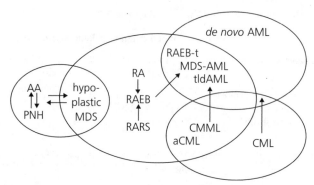

Fig. 4.1 The myelodysplastic syndrome overlap syndromes.

The MDS overlap syndromes

MDS shares common features with other stem cell disorders such as aplastic anaemia, paroxysmal nocturnal haemoglobinuria, atypical chronic myeloid leukaemia, and trilineage dysplasia AML. Progression from one category to another may be observed (Fig. 4.1).

Hypoplastic MDS, defined as dysplastic haemopoiesis associated with BM cellularity of less than 25–30%, is not a subgroup in any classification system. It shares features in common with aplastic anaemia and paroxysmal nocturnal haemoglobinuria. It is an important subgroup to identify, as patients respond well to immunosuppressive treatment with anti-lymphocyte globulin.

Clinical features of MDS

The syndrome usually presents in older patients with a median age at presentation of 60–75 years. Macrocytic anaemia with a normal B12, folate, or isolated cytopenias may exist for years prior to the patient developing symptoms. Recurrent infections, bleeding, and symptoms of anaemia secondary to marrow failure are the commonest presenting symptoms.

On examination, pallor, bruising, splenomegaly, and sometimes lymphadenopathy may be evident.

Association with vasculitis, pyoderma gangrenosum, relapsing polychondritis, and acute neutrophilic dermatitis has been described. Pleural and pericardial effusions may occur with CMML.

Peripheral blood and bone marrow features

Dysplastic morphology (Table 4.4) is evident in both peripheral blood and bone marrow. These changes are not entirely specific to MDS and can on

Table 4.4 Morphological abnormalities in myelodysplastic syndrome

Cell lineage	Peripheral blood	Bone marrow
Erythroid	Anaemia Macrocytes Dimorphic red blood cells Anisopoikilocytosis Schistocytes Basophilic stippling Normoblasts	Megaloblasts Cytoplasmic vacuolation Ringed sideroblasts Polyploidy Multinuclearity Nuclear budding Internuclear bridging Basophilic stippling Pyknosis Erythroid hyperplasia or hypoplasia
Granulocyte	Neutropenia Hypogranular/agranular neutrophils Pseudo-pelger neutrophils Abnormal nuclear segmentation Ring form nucleus	Granulocytic hyperplasia Abnormal nuclear lobulation Abnormal cytoplasmic granulation
Megakaryocyte	Thrombocytopenia Occasional thrombocytosis Giant platelets Hypo or hypergranular platelets Megakaryocyte fragments	Mono/hypolobated megakaryocytes Abnormal nuclear lobulation Micromegakaryocytes Reduced cytoplasmic granulation
Monocytic	Abnormal nuclear shape Increased cytoplasmic basophilia	Promonocytes may be increased

Blasts	Type I
	  Small Mononuclear blasts
	  With scanty agranular cytoplasm
	Type II
	  Sparsely granular blasts
	  Auer rods (RAEB-t)	

occasions be identified in acutely ill patients, alcoholism, HIV infection, hypothyroidism, and post-chemotherapy.

Marrow histology shows disruption of the normal bone marrow architecture with displacement of megakaryocytes and erythroid islands from their normal inter-trabecular location to a para-trabecular one. Likewise, islands of myeloid precursors form in an inter-trabecular area and are termed ALIP (abnormal localization of immature precursors). These are a hallmark of MDS and are usually associated with poor outcome in patients with refractory anaemia and refractory anaemia with ring sideroblasts. Cellularity of the marrow in MDS is normal or hypercellular in most cases. In a third of cases, the marrow may be hypocellular and, if less than 30%, is considered hypoplastic MDS.

Reticulin is mildly to moderately increased in MDS marrows, however in 15% of patients there is marked fibrosis. There is a clinical overlap in this subset with myeloproliferative disorders. The marrow is frequently hyper-cellular and small megakaryocytes with hypolobated nuclei predominate. Clinically, patients may have organomegaly, pancytopenia, and dysplastic morphology. There may be a history of prior mutagenic exposure.

Prognostic factors

The FAB classification determines prognosis to some extent and has been the basis of several prognostic-scoring systems. Patients with RA and RARS have a median survival of 4.2 and 6.9 years, respectively, and an 8–12% risk of leukaemic transformation. The survival is significantly shorter in RAEB and RAEB-t with median of 11 and 5 months, respectively. Rates of leukaemic progression are also higher at 44% and 60%, respectively.

The International Prognostic Scoring System (Table 4.5) was generated by a combination of weighted variables derived from a multivariate analysis of clinical and laboratory features of 816 untreated primary MDS patients.[8] The most significant independent variables for determining survival and leukaemic evolution were, in order of significance: BM blast percentage, kary-otype, and the number of cytopenias. Combining these identified four major prognostic groups. It has been validated against other scoring systems and accurately predicts outcomes within FAB subgroups.

Advanced age and secondary disease are adverse prognostic factors. Other prognostic factors include:

♦ BM blast percentage: with less than 5% being associated with a good prog-nosis, as opposed to an intermediate-poor prognosis if these are greater than 10%.

♦ Normal cytogenetics, isolated del 5q, 20q, -Y with normal residual metaphases have a good prognosis, whereas other cytogenetic abnormalit-ies or karyotypic evolution predict a poor outcome.

♦ Cytopenias of more than one lineage, raised LDH, peripheral blood blasts, and severe morphological dysplasia are poor prognostic features. ALIP, reti-culin fibrosis, increased microvessel density; increased BM CD34 positive cells with CD34+ cell aggregates are adverse histological features. *In vitro* cultures with increased cluster to colony ratio or no growth also forecast a poorer prognosis, as compared to a good one with normal *in vitro* culture.

♦ Molecular evidence of the N- or K-RAS mutation, FMS mutation, p53 mutation/deletion, increased wilm's tumour (WT1) expression and of p15INK4B gene hypermethylation are linked to a poor prognosis.

Table 4.5 The international prognostic scoring system (IPSS)

Prognostic variable	Score 0	Score 0.5	Score 1.0	Score 1.5	Score 2.0
BM blast %	<5	5–10	–	11–20	21–30
Karyotype	Good	Intermediate	Poor		
Cytopenias	0/1	2/3			

	<60 years	>60 years	<70 years	>70 years
Median survival (years): IPSS score				
Low	11.8	4.8	9	3.9
Intermediate-1	5.2	2.7	4.4	2.4
Intermediate-2	1.8	1.1	1.3	1.2
High	0.3	0.5	0.4	0.4

Risk groups: Low: score 0

        Intermediate −1: score 0.5–1

        Intermediate −2: score 1.5–2

        High: >2.5

Karyotype: Good: normal, del 5q, 20q-, -Y

        Intermediate: other abnormalities

        Poor: complex (>3 abnormalities) or chromosome 7 abnormalities

Management

This is often complicated by the advanced age of patients and that they often have pre-existing disease unrelated to MDS. A 'wait and watch' policy is prudent for many patients. The aim of the treatment is to reduce morbidity and mortality, whilst maintaining an acceptable quality of life. This is often achieved by supportive care.

Supportive care

Supportive care is the mainstay of management of patients with good prognosis MDS and in those with poor prognosis disease where clinical factors preclude intensive therapy. In early MDS, the decision to transfuse with blood products is based on symptoms and blood counts. When, however, palliation and improving quality of life is the main focus of care, blood product administration is guided by symptoms such as dyspnoea and bleeding, rather than haemaglobin (Hb) level and platelet counts.

Anaemia

Symptomatic anaemia is the commonest clinical problem in low-risk MDS and can lead to significant morbidity. Blood transfusions should be considered for such people and symptoms should be the trigger for a transfuion rather than Hb concentration. This treatment is commonly associated with complications such as transfusion reactions, immunomodulation, and iron overload. It is an expensive and time-consuming procedure with patients having to attend hospital frequently for prolonged periods of time.

Studies in cancer patients have demonstrated a positive correlation between increases in Hb concentration and improvements in quality of life, particularly when the Hb rose from 11g/dl to 12g/dl, suggesting that even mildly anaemic patients who are not currently transfused may benefit from efforts to increase haemoglobin levels.

Iron chelation therapy with desferrioxamine is recommended for patients who have received more than 25 units of blood transfusion

Erythropoietin: recombinant human erythropoietin can improve anaemia in 20% of patient with MDS. This response is confined to patients with serum EPO level <200 units/l, minimal pre-treatment blood transfusion requirements and a FAB subtype other than RARS.

The co-administration of G-CSF or GM-CSF is additive in enhancing the erythroid response to erythropoietin[9] and reduces transfusion requirements in up to 52% of cases with RARS.

Novel erythropoiesis-stimulating protein (NESP, darbepoietin-α) stimulates erythropoiesis by the same mechanism as EPO but is biochemically distinct. It has a three-fold greater serum half-life and therefore requires less frequent administration. It is effective in maintaining Hb levels in chronic renal failure and may be effective in the treatment of anaemia in MDS. It is not in regular clinical use at present.

Neutropenia

This may be ameliorated by the administration of granulocyte colony stimulating factor (G-CSF) or granulocyte macrophage colony stimulating factor (GM-CSF). The response rate may improve by the addition of the differentiating agent all-trans retinoic acid (ATRA). However, randomized trials have failed to demonstrate any positive effect on survival. Administration of the multipotent haemopoietic cytokines interleukin-3 (IL-3) and IL-6, alone or in combination with G-CSF/GM-CSF have been disappointing and are frequently associated with significant toxicity.

Bleeding disorders

Prolonged bleeding in MDS due to platelet dysfunction or thrombocytopenia responds to treatment with platelet transfusions. The former should be considered if patients are undergoing surgery. Further discussion of this topic will be found in Chapter 12.

Disease-modifying agents

Trophic and differentiating agents

Hypermethylation of the p15 INK4B gene, with consequent silencing, is considered pathogenic in MDS. 5-Azacytidine and 5-aza-2'-deoxycytidine are pyrimidine analogues that inhibit DNA methyltransferase activity and could improve myelodysplastic haemopoiesis by reversing aberrant gene methylation and permitting cellular differentiation.

5-Azacytidine has been demonstrated to be a potent inducer of differentiation in myeloid leukaemia cell lines. It has so far been tried in high-risk patients with up to 63% demonstrating improvements in blood counts and/or cytogenetic responses. Kornblith et al.,[10] in a large, prospective, randomized, phase III study found that 5-azacytidine treated patients showed a significantly lower probability of AML transformation, delayed time to leukaemic progression, or death and improved quality of life compared to the observation arm. A similar world-wide phase III trial is due to commence in early 2003.

Sodium phenylbutyrate is another potent differentiating agent that appears to alter transcriptional regulation of gene expression by inhibiting DNA methylation and histone de-acetylation. Of patients with MDS or non-proliferative AML, 63% in a phase I trial demonstrated improvements in peripheral counts following sodium phenylbutyrate administration. Currently it is an experimental agent.

Amifostine is a DNA-binding aminothiol, which enhances in vitro growth of normal and MDS progenitors whilst reducing the number of bone marrow CD34+ cells undergoing apoptosis. Altogether, 83% haematological response rates in patients with improved in vitro progenitor colony growth have been shown using intravenous Amifostine. The addition of growth factor or agents that suppress cytokine-mediated cell death, such as pentoxyfylline, ciprofloxacin, and dexamethasone, was shown to yield improved results by Raza et al.[11] Unfortunately their findings have not been universally replicated and it cannot currently be recommended for use in MDS.

Immunomodulatory agents

The suppression of haemopoiesis in MDS, like that in PNH and aplastic anaemia (AA), is thought to be immune mediated. Cases of hypoplastic MDS also have frequent overlap with AA and PNH. This has prompted the use of anti-thymocyte globulin[12] and cyclosporin, which have produced sustained haematological responses in 44% and 84% cases, respectively. The presence of a PNH clone, BM hypocellularity, and less than 5% BM blasts, are positive predictors of response to immunomodulation.

Chemotherapeutic agents

Low-intensity chemotherapy

Suppression of dysplastic clones without haematological toxicity may be achieved by the use of low-dose chemotherapy. Trials with low-dose cytarabine yielded response in 10–25% of MDS/MDS-AML patients, although no survival benefit over the use of supportive therapy alone has been shown. Similar results have been seen with low-dose anthracyclines and homoharringtonine. Low-dose melphalan may produce durable remissions in up to one-third of elderly patients. Topotecan, a topoisomerase-I inhibitor, has produced a response in 43% of patients with advanced MDS or CMML.

The combination of cytarabine and topotecan may yield better responses, especially in MDS associated with chromosome 5/7 abnormalities.

The use of low-dose cytarabine, idarubicin, and thioguanine is not routinely recommended in MDS, however the role of topotecan in intensive-combination regimes appears encouraging.

Intensive chemotherapy

Patients with advanced MDS/MDS-AML have a poorer response to chemotherapy compared with *de novo* AML. Most patients relapse within 12 months of attaining remisssion. This may be due to advanced patient age; attendant co-morbidity prolonged chemotherapy induced aplasia, which resulted in increased regimen-related toxicity. Chemotherapy resistance is also common due to the presence of unbalanced karyotypic abnormalities, blasts that express a stem cell phenotype, and over-expression of p glycoproteins. The addition of quinine may improve survival in those expressing multi-drug resistance phenotypes.

Treatment with fludarabine, cytarabine G-CSF (FLAG), and FLAG with idarubicin (FLAG-Ida) has been encouraging and may be most beneficial to MDS patients with a poor prognosis karyotype.

Autologous stem cell transplantation

The demonstration of the ability to harvest polyclonal stem cells from MDS patients has made this a feasible option for patients. Trials in those in complete remission (CR) following induction chemotherapy have shown a 38% 2-year overall survival, 33% disease-free survival, and relapse rates of 53%. Outcomes were significantly better in patients younger than 40 years and in those with good or intermediate risk karyotype at diagnosis. However, a significant number of patients do not undergo autologous transplants due to poor performance status, failure to achieve CR, early relapse, or inadequate stem cell harvests.

Allogeneic stem cell transplantation

The fact that intensive chemotherapy does not achieve prolonged disease-free survival in patients with MDS, has made it necessary to search for other means of a cure. To date, allogeneic bone marrow transplantation is the only means of a potential cure for MDS.[13]

As MDS is caused by expansion of an abnormal clone of pluripotent stem cells, myeloablative therapy can be used to eradicate the abnormal clone followed by establishment of normal haemopoiesis by the allograft.

More recently it has become clear that the effects of a bone marrow transplant are not entirely explained by pre-transplant chemotherapy or radiation and that patients with graft versus host disease had a lower rate of relapse. The phenomenon is thought to be due to the immune reactivity of allogeneic T lymphocytes against leukaemic cells and has been termed the 'graft versus leukaemic' effect.

The identification of this effect has led to the emergence of 'reduced intensity conditioning' allografts (RIC-allografts) or non-myeloablative stem cell therapy.[14]

These reduce the intensity of pre-transplant conditioning chemotherapy balanced by increasing the level of immunosuppression to harness the graft-versus-leukaemia effect. Comparison between this and conventional allogeneic stem cell transplantation in patients with MDS has shown that it is feasible, that patients with a greater median age (48.5 years versus 37.5 years) and those with pre-existing organ damage can undergo such a transplant.

Using the fludarabine, busulphan Campath protocol and cyclosporin/ methotrexate GvHD prophylaxis, full donor engraftment was achieved in 100% of cases transplanted in CR. The duration of neutropenia was diminished with a reduction in the supportive care necessary. The rate of GvHD was less and at 1–13 months follow-up, 80% of the patients were in continuing CR.

Because of the variable outcome of patients with MDS, patient selection for allogeneic bone marrow transplantation is a critical issue. Young patients (less than 40 years) with MDS and an HLA identical sibling donor should undergo early transplantation before the advent of cytopenias, life-threatening complications, or disease progression, which can adversely affect or prevent transplantation. Matched unrelated donor transplants were previously restricted to those under 35 years with poor risk MDS but with the advent of RIC, transplants (less toxic) are being extended to older patients (upto 60 years).

Patients with RAEB or RAEB-t, marked cytopenias (neutrophils $<0.5 \times 10^9/1$ or platelet count $<20 \times 10^9/1$), and/or poor prognosis cytogenetics are potential allo-BMT recipients, as their average survival is less than one year.

Improved outcomes following transplantation are seen in those who are younger, have a shorter disease duration, primary MDS, good risk cytogenetics, low IPSS score, BM blasts up to 10%, HLA-compatible donors, and are in CR. Post-allo-BMT 5-year disease-free survival from 32 to 52% have been seen. However, the presence of increased numbers of blasts, high-risk cytogenetics, prolonged disease duration, and older age increase the risk of relapse. Interstitial pneumonia and GvHD contribute to decreased long-term survival in transplant recipients.

Novel agents

Arsenic trioxide, farnesyl transferase inhibitors (currently in a phase II trial in the UK), the tyrosine kinase inhibitor Imatinib, soluble tumour necrosis factor receptor (Enbrel), chimaeric anti-TNF, a monoclonal antibody (Infliximab), and antangiogenesis agents such as thalidomide, SU5416, and anti-vascular endothelial growth factor (VEGF) antibodies are undergoing clinical trials in MDS.

Concluding remarks

The myelodysplastic syndromes are a spectrum of pre-leukaemic disorders that manifest predominantly in the elderly and can have a prolonged course. Patients require regular monitoring for evidence of disease progression, infection, and cytopenias, which may be ameliorated with good supportive care. Decisions regarding intervention with high-dose chemotherapy or bone marrow transplantation should be guided by the IPSS scoring system. The timing of such intervention in the younger patient needs to be balanced between the risk of progression and their current life situation. In the elderly, who are the great majority of patients, antecedent medical conditions and performance status frequently make the above strategies inappropriate. In this situation, palliation of symptoms and appropriate supportive care are the mainstays of treatment. Particular support is also required when the disease progresses or transforms to AML. New drugs and the advent of reduced intensity conditioning transplants offer the hope of cure to an increased number of patients.

References

1 Bennett, J. M., Catovsky, D., Daniel, M. T. *et al.* (1982). Proposals for the classification of the myelodysplastic syndromes. *Br J Haematol*, **51**, 189.
2 Saso, R., Kulkarni, S., Mitchell, P. *et al.* (2000). Secondary myelodysplastic syndrome/acute myeloid leukaemia following mitoxantrone-based therapy for breast carcinoma. *Br J Cancer*, **83**, 91–94.

3 Pedersen-Bjergaard, J., Andersen, M. K., and Christiansen, D. H. (2000). Therapy-related acute myeloid leukaemia and myelodysplasia after high dose chemotherapy and autologous stem cell transplantation (review). *Blood*, **95**, 3273–9.

4 Morrow, N. L. (1990). The industrial production and use of 1,3-butadiene (review). *Environ Health Perspect*, **86**, 7–8.

5 Raza, A. (1998). Hypothesis: myelodysplastic syndromes may have an infectious aetiology (review). *Int J Haematol*, **68**, 245–56.

6 Parker, J., Mufti, G. J., Rasool, F. *et al.* (2000). The role of apoptosis, proliferation and Bcl-2-related proteins in the myelodysplastic syndromes and acute myeloid leukaemia secondary to MDS. *Blood*, **96**, 3932–8.

7 Harris, N. L., Jaffe, E. S., Diebold, J. *et al.* (1999). World Health Organisation classification of neoplastic diseases of the haemopoietic and lymphoid tissues: report of the Clinical Advisory Committee meeting-Airlie House, Virginia, November 1997. *J Clin Oncol*, **17**, 3835–49.

8 Greenberg, P., Cox, C., Lebeau, M. M. *et al.* (1997). International scoring system for evaluating prognosis in myelodysplastic syndromes. *Blood*, **89**, 2079–88.

9 Hellstrom Lindberg, E., Ahlgren, T., Beguin, Y. *et al.* (1998). Treatment of anemia in myelodysplastic syndromes with granulocyte colony stimulating factor plus erythropoietin: results from a randomised phase II study and long term follow-up of 71 patients. *Blood*, **92**, 68–75.

10 Kornblith, A. B., Herndon, J. E., Lewis, R. *et al.* (2002). Impact of Azacytidine on the quality of life of patients with Myelodysplastic Syndrome treated in a randomised Phase III trial: a cancer and leukaemia study group B study. *JCO*, **10**, 2441–52.

11 Raza, A., Qawi, H., Lisak, L. *et al.* (2000). Patients with myelodysplastic syndromes benefit form palliative therapy with amifostine, pentoxifylline, and ciprofloxacin with or without dexamethasone. *Blood*, **95**, 1580–7.

12 Killick, S. B., Marsh, J. C., Cavenagh, J. D. *et al.* (1999). Antithymocyte globulin for the treatment of patients with low risk myelodysplastic syndromes. *Blood*, **94**, 1371.

13 Deeg, H. J., Shulman, H. M., Anderson, J. (2000). Allogeneic and syngeneic marrow transplantation for myelodysplastic syndrome in patients 55 to 66 years of age. *Blood*, **95**, 1188–94.

14 Slavin, S., Nagler, A., Naparstek, E. *et al.* (1998). Non-myeloablative stem cell transplantation and cell therapy as an alternative to conventional bone marrow transplantation with lethal cytoreduction for the treatment of malignant and nonmalignant haematologic diseases. *Blood*, **91**, 756–63.

Chapter 5

Bone marrow and peripheral blood stem cell transplantation

Helen Balsdon and Jenny I. O. Craig

Introduction

This chapter aims to give an overview of stem cell transplantation. It will explain the terminology involved, the different types of transplantation, and the common problems associated with this treatment.

Background

Haematopoietic stem cell transplantation allows the delivery of high doses of chemotherapy and radiotherapy to patients, overcoming the resultant marrow aplasia by infusing stem cells (either from a donor or the patient's own previously stored cells), which repopulate the haematopoietic system.

The aim of stem cell transplantation is usually cure and hence it is performed when conventional, less toxic standard treatments are unlikely to result in long-term control of the underlying disease.

The disease-specific chapters have discussed the role of transplantation in various haematological malignancies. However, transplantation is also used to treat non-malignant diseases, e.g. some congenital immune deficiency disorders, and genetic disorders such as thalassaemia, although these are less common indications.

Types of transplants

A transplant can be defined as the infusion of haematopoietic stem (or progenitor) cells after chemotherapy, with or without radiotherapy. Transplants can be categorized according to

- the type of donor:
  - autologous
  - sibling allogeneic
  - volunteer unrelated
  - syngeneic

- ◆ the source of the stem cells:
  - • bone marrow
  - • peripheral blood
  - • cord blood.

Autologous transplant

In autologous transplantation the donor and recipient is the same person. Stem cells are collected at a time prior to the transplant, usually when there is evidence of remission, and stored at low temperatures (cryopreserved).

During the transplant, high-dose treatment in the form of chemotherapy, with or without radiotherapy (called conditioning), is given with the aim of killing any residual malignant cells in the body. The stem cells are thawed and infused through a central venous line into the bloodstream and 'home' to the bone marrow. After 2–4 weeks the white cells, platelets, and red cells will show signs of recovery as the stem cells 'engraft'. This procedure is not without risk; the treatment-related mortality (TRM) depends on the source of stem cells used. If peripheral blood stem cells (PBSC) are infused, the TRM is approximately 3–5% as the blood counts take less time to recover (2–3 weeks) compared to bone marrow stem cells (3–4 weeks), when the TRM may be up to 10%.[1] The risks are related to marrow aplasia, including infection and haemorrhage, and to organ damage from conditioning treatment. This procedure is suitable for patients of less than 65 years of age and from whom stem cells can be harvested. Disease relapse after autologous transplant remains a risk.

Sibling allogeneic transplant

In sibling allogeneic transplants, stem cells are collected from a human leuko-cyte antigen (HLA) compatible brother or sister. There is only a one in four chance of a patient having an HLA-identical sibling and only about 10% of eligible patients will therefore be able to have this type of transplant. As in the autologous setting, conditioning is followed by stem cell infusion, however as the graft is derived from a donor, immunosuppresion must be given to allow engraftment and prevent graft versus host disease (see below).

As the risks involved in allogeneic transplantation increase with age, this treat-ment is often restricted to those under 50 years. Toxicity results not only from conditioning and marrow aplasia but also from other complications related to allogeneic transplantation, such as acute graft versus host disease (GvHD), veno-occlusive disease (VOD) of the liver, and interstitial pneumonitis (see below). The transplant-related mortality is around 20%. In addition to receiving disease-free stem cells, there may be an immunological 'graft versus leukaemia' effect of an allogeneic transplant that can reduce the risks of disease relapse.

Volunteer-unrelated allogeneic transplant

As most patients requiring allogeneic transplants do not have a sibling donor, volunteer bone marrow donor registries were established internationally to provide a pool of available HLA-typed donors. Volunteer unrelated donor (VUD) transplants are performed in a similar way to sibling allogeneic transplants, however the risk of graft versus host disease is greater, with a resultant increase in transplant-related mortality of around 30–50% in older patients. These are generally offered to patients less than 35 years old.

Syngeneic transplant

Syngeneic transplantation is uncommon, whereby stem cells are collected from a genetically identical twin. In many respects, although this type of transplant uses a donor to provide stem cells, it is similar to an autologous transplant. There is little graft versus leukaemia effect and a greater chance of relapse than in sibling allogeneic transplantation.

Cord blood transplant

Cord blood transplantation is an experimental procedure. Cord blood contains stem cells and it was hoped that these would be immunologically naïve and thus reduce the risks of graft versus host disease seen in unrelated donor transplants. Volunteer cord banks were established to increase the number of different HLA-typed donations available. The numbers of stem cells present however may only be sufficient to transplant a child.

The type of transplant procedure performed is generally the least toxic required to achieve cure or long-term disease control. Decision-making about the type of procedure is based upon type of disease, age of recipient, physical and, to some extent, psychological well-being of the recipient and in the allogeneic setting, donor availability. The risks of transplant compared to the potential benefits are considered with the patients during the pre-transplant assessment phase.

Collection of stem cells

Stem cells may be collected from bone marrow or blood.

Bone marrow harvesting

During a bone marrow harvest the patient or donor is given a general anaesthetic and placed prone. Up to 20 ml/kg of bone marrow is aspirated from the right and left posterior iliac crests (rarely also the anterior iliac crests) and transferred to collection bags for processing by the stem cell laboratory.

Peripheral blood stem cell harvesting

Stem cells are first mobilized from the marrow into the blood and then collected by leukapheresis using a cell separator. Mobilization of PBSC into the blood occurs as the white blood cell count recovers after myelosuppressive chemotherapy, aided by an approximately 8–10 day course of a growth factor such as granulocyte colony stimulating factor (G-CSF). In patients or in healthy donors in whom chemotherapy is not appropriate, a 4–5 day course of growth factor alone can be given.

The transplant procedure

Conditioning

Conditioning refers to the chemotherapy and/or radiotherapy given prior to stem cell infusion. In allogeneic transplants, immunosuppressive therapy is also started. The aim of conditioning is to destroy residual disease, to provide physical space for the new stem cells to grow (although the need for this is controversial), and in the allogeneic setting to ensure an adequate level of immunosuppression to allow engraftment. These have predictable toxicities (see below).

There are many different types of conditioning regimens and the choice depends upon the underlying disease. Chemotherapy is used in most regimens. The 'gold standard' regimen in the allogeneic setting is cyclophosphamide and total body irradiation (TBI). In view of the lack of availability of radiotherapy facilities and the desire to reduce toxicity, chemotherapy only regimens such as busulphan combined with cyclophosphamide, which is effective in myeloid malignancies, have been developed. Although radiotherapy was originally given at one treatment sitting, fractionation of the dose was introduced to reduce the incidence and severity of complications. 10–15 Gy is typically given in 5–8 fractions over 3–5 days.

More recently, adjustments to the conditioning regimen in order to reduce toxicity further (called non-myeloablative or mini-transplants) have been made in allogeneic and unrelated donor settings. These experimental transplants rely on the immune component (graft versus leukaemia effect) of transplantation to destroy disease, rather than high doses of chemo/radiotherapy. Such transplants are less toxic and can be performed in a wider range of patients, however their long-term effects on disease have not yet been established and relapse remains a significant risk.

Side-effects of conditioning

Potential problems at this stage result from acute chemo/radiotherapy induced organ damage. As the onset may be delayed, generally recipients feel relatively well during the conditioning phase. Immediate side-effects of chemotherapy include nausea and vomiting, diarrhoea and constipation. Immediate TBI complications are similar, but also include syncope (some radiotherapy centres administer the doses in a semi-standing position), fevers and chill, parotitis (which may be painful), increased skin sensitivity, and occasionally skin reactions and early mucositis.

Stem cell infusion

Stem cells are infused 24–48 h following the end of conditioning via a central line. Complications include nausea, vomiting, chills, fevers, (usually related to the cryoprotectant DMSO).

Engraftment and the first 100 days

Engraftment occurs when there is evidence of recovery of haematopoiesis. This is often defined as the days taken from stem cell infusion until neutrophils are greater than $0.5 \times 10^9/l$ and platelets greater than $50 \times 10^9/l$. Examples of engraftment time are shown in Table 5.1.

Potential early complications include bone marrow failure, gastro-intestinal and other direct organ toxicities, acute graft versus host disease.

Bone marrow failure results in anaemia, thrombocytopaenia, and neutropenia. Supportive care of the first two relies on blood product support. Cellular products are irradiated to prevent transfusion-associated GvHD. Previously, cytomegalovirus (CMV) sero-negative transplants were given products from donors screened negative for the virus. However, quality assured laboratory based leukodepletion of blood products is considered equivalent to donor screening and is widely available. Anaemia is managed by administering packed red cells to maintain the haemoglobin above 10 g/dl. Equally, thrombocytopaenia can be managed by prophylactic platelet

Table 5.1 Comparison of autologous PBSCT, BMT, and allogeneic BMT

	Auto PBSC	Auto BMT	AlloBMT
Neutrophils $>0.5 \times 10^9/l$	11 days	22 days	24.5 days
Platelets $>50 \times 10^9/l$	13.5 days	32 days	33 days
Days until discharge after infusion	16.5	25	26
Platelet transfusions required	3 units	10 units	9 units

transfusions above $10 \times 10^9/l$, or higher should the recipient be febrile or actively bleeding.

The infection risk in the autologous setting results mainly from neutropenia and the disruption of the normal barriers to infection, such as the skin or gastro-intestinal tract which allows bacterial invasion.

In the allogeneic setting there is the additional immunosuppression associated with drugs such as cyclosporin used to prevent GvHD. This affects T-cell function and can be present for weeks or months, especially if GvHD develops, resulting in an increased risk from viral and fungal pathogens

Nearly all patients undergoing transplant will develop fever whilst neutropenic. Only about 40% will be associated with a documented microbial infection. With the use of in-dwelling central catheters, the commonest organisms isolated are Gram-positive, skin-related bacteria such as coagulase negative staphylococci. Gram-negative sepsis is less common but life-threatening. Prevention of infection includes good patient hygiene, careful hand washing by staff and visitors, low antimicrobial diets, physical environment control, and antimicrobial prophylaxis, e.g. quinolones. The transplant unit will institute early therapy of fever in neutropenic patients with broad spectrum antibiotics appropriate for the local antimicrobial sensitivities of candidate organisms.

Other infections include fungi, especially *Candida* and *Aspergillus*, which can be found in up to one-third of transplants. These infections can have a high mortality and require therapy with amphotericin-based compounds, including the less toxic lipid formulations. Prevention of fungal infections includes the use of fluconazole or itraconazole. Infection rates with *Candida* have decreased but *Aspergillus* and other moulds resistant to fluconazole are an increasing problem.[2]

In the early post-transplant phase, herpes simplex virus may reactivate, contributing to oral pain. Aciclovir prophylaxis can help prevent this. CMV is a major risk in the allogeneic and unrelated-donor setting. CMV infection usually results from reactivation when either the recipient or donor carries this virus. The most serious infections, including interstitial pneumonitis with a mortality of 85%, occur when a seropositive donor receives stem cells from a seronegative recipient. This emphasizes the importance of control of the virus by donor immunity. The drug ganciclovir can be used as treatment or as prophylaxis against CMV reactivation. Often patients are closely monitored by blood PCR and treated should this become positive.

Pneumocystis is a protozoan parasite that also causes interstitial pneumonia. Prevention of infection is with co-trimoxazole prophylaxis from engraftment until 6–12 months after transplant.

Gastro-intestinal disturbances

Many patients experience nausea and vomiting due to the conditioning regimen and other drugs, which in turn results in fluid and electrolyte disturbance. Anti-emetic prophylaxis and therapy is important (see Chapters 6 and 8).

Predictably, conditioning causes mucositis, oesophagitis, gastroduodenitis, and widespread mucosal damage resulting in pain, poor nutritional intake, and diarrhoea. Analgesia (see Chapter X) and nutritional supplementation (parenteral or via the GI tract) may be required. These changes may be accompanied by viral or fungal infection, which will need specific therapy. Gastro-intestinal changes may last for up to 6 weeks. Diarrhoea, in addition to being a direct toxic effect of conditioning, can result from bacterial/viral infection. The serious complication of neutropenic enterocolitis (typhlitis) results in massive dilatation of the bowel with the risk of perforation, sepsis, and mortality. Pseudomenbranous colitis from *C. difficile* toxin can present a similar clinical picture. It usually responds to oral metronidazole or vancomycin. Acute GvHD affects the GI tract presenting as green watery diarrhoea (see below).

Organ toxicity

High-dose therapy can be toxic to many vital organs. The potential complications are discussed below.

Renal and urinary tract

Acute renal failure may potentially result from pre-renal causes (sepsis, bleeding, dehydration) directly from conditioning regimens, or from drugs (cyclosporin, antibiotics). Fluid and electrolyte balance is closely monitored. The haemolytic uraemic syndrome with red cell fragmentation, haemolysis, and renal impairment is recognized after transplant, contributed to by cyclosporin. Haemorrhagic cystitis may arise as a result of cyclophosphamide, radiation, or viral infection. This can be mild or extremely painful requiring bladder irrigation.

Pulmonary system

Pulmonary complications occur in 20–40% of transplants and are one of the commonest causes of death in the early post-transplant period.[3] Causes include infection (bacterial, viral, fungal) fluid overload, cardiac failure, bleeding, and other non-infectious complications. Idiopathic interstitial pneumonitis has a peak incidence between 30 and 100 days after the transplant, presenting as breathlessness, dry cough, hypoxia, and pulmonary infiltrates on X-ray. The mortality is high—approximately 50% will die. CT scanning and bronchoscopy are useful investigations. Ventilatory support and intensive care may be necessary.

Cardiovascular complications

Cardiac complications occur in approximately 25% of transplant patients. These include complications such as cardiac failure, endocarditis, hyper/hypotension, and ECG changes. Life-threatening cardiac complications occur in 5–10% of patients who have received cyclophosphamide-based conditioning regimens, presenting usually as congestive cardiac failure 3 weeks after conditioning.

Hepatic complications

Abnormalities in liver function tests are common after transplantation, often related to drugs but also to sepsis. More significant is acute graft versus host disease (see below) and veno-occulsive disease (VOD). Hepatic VOD is a serious complication resulting from damage to the endothelium of small intrahepatic venules with obstruction and hepatocyte destruction. This classically presents in the first 3 weeks after transplant with jaundice, tender hepatomegaly, abdominal distention from ascites with resultant weight gain. VOD occurs in 10–60% of patients with an average mortality of 30–40%. Risk factors include abnormal transaminases pre-transplant. Diagnosis is difficult and predominantly clinical. Treatment of the disease rests with good fluid and electrolyte balance. Successful treatment is not well established but anti-thrombotic/thrombolytic agents such as tPA, defibreotide, and anticoagulation have been used although results are variable.[4]

Central nervous system complications

Altered consciousness or fits may occur as a consequence of metabolic disturbances, infections, or drugs, as above. Thrombocytopenia may result in an intracerebral bleed.

More specifically, a somnolence syndrome, related to TBI and manifesting as a period of drowsiness/tiredness and nausea, approximately 6–8 weeks after transplant is common, especially in children and young adults. Many patients will only feel increased tiredness for about 2 weeks; others will also experience nausea and vomiting, dizziness and headaches. Management relies on rest and maintaining a good fluid intake. Occasionally steroids are helpful, if the syndrome is severe.

Graft versus host disease

There are two types of GvHD: acute (occurring in the first 100 days after allogeneic transplant); and chronic (occurring from 3 months onwards)—see below.

Acute GvHD

Acute GvHD occurs in up to 40% of recipients of matched allogeneic transplants. It manifests as a skin rash, jaundice, or diarrhoea. It is caused by immunologically competent T-lymphocytes, infused with the donor stem cells, recognizing the recipient as 'foreign' and mounting a reaction targeted at:

- *skin* causing a rash initially on the palms and soles extending to the whole skin;
- *liver* bile duct epithelium with intrahepatic cholestasis and hepatocyte damage;
- *intestines* causing green diarrhoea, abdominal pain and paralytic ileus.

Acute GvHD is graded I–IV depending on the severity. Survival from grade I is good but the mortality from grades III and IV is very high. The risk of GvHD increases with age and is the major limiting factor in allogeneic transplantation.

The diagnosis of acute GvHD is clinical or by biopsy of the affected area. First-line therapy is steroid treatment (topical or parenteral depending upon the affected site or stage/grade of the disease) to suppress the immune function. The mortality of steroid-resistant GvHD is 80%. In view of the mortality and morbidity of GvHD, prevention is an important approach. This is done by HLA matching donor and recipient, immunosuppression with drugs such as cyclosporin and methotrexate, and *in vivo* or *in vitro* T-cell depletion of the graft.

Late complications

Complications after 3 months include infection, chronic GvHD, infertility, and endocrine dysfunction, relapse, psychological morbidity, and secondary malignancies.

Infection

Late infections can be a major cause of mortality in this period due to functional hyposplenism or continued immunosuppression in allogeneic transplants, particularly those with chronic GvHD. The combined immunodeficiency affecting B and T cells may take months or even years to recover. The most common types of late infections include encapsulated organisms such as pneumococcal infections and viral infections, e.g. CMV, respiratory viruses, herpes zoster (shingles). Patients should be made aware of these risks and any late infection should be reported and treated promptly. Re-vaccination against tetanus, diphtheria, polio (inactivated), pnuemococci, influenza, and

HIB should be given usually between 6 and 12 months post-transplant, as immunity to these organisms is lost.

Chronic GvHD

Chronic GvHD (cGvHD) is the most common late complication of allogeneic stem cell transplantation, occurring in more than 50% of recipients. Older patients, those receiving a peripheral blood stem cell graft, or an unrelated transplant are more at risk. cGvHD occurs after 100 days, the median time of onset in sibling allogeneic recipients is 200 days post-transplant. It can occur without antecedent GvHD (*de novo*) progressively from aGvHD (worst prognosis) or after a quiescent period. The syndrome resembles an autoimmune disease, with a lack of immune tolerance and a central role for T cells, which are reactive against the recipient. Both alloreactive and autoreactive T cells appear important in the pathogenesis, but this is still not fully elucidated.

Diagnosis rests on clinical suspicion confirmed by biopsy of affected sites. The extent of disease is then determined and staged as either limited (localized to either skin or liver dysfunction or both) or extensive (as limited but with oral, eye or other organ involvement).[5]

The manifestations of chronic GvHD are listed in Table 5.2. Poor prognostic features include skin involvement of $>50\%$, thrombocytopenia $<100 \times 10^9/l$, progressive onset, and a poor performance status.

Table 5.2 Clinical presentations of chronic GvHD

Organ	Clinical features
Skin	Sclerodermatous (thin tight) or lichenoid (red rash) changes
Hair	Thinning or alopecia
Eyes	Dry, risk of corneal abrasion
Mouth	Dry, sensitive to heat and spice, white plaques cheeks tongue (lichen planus), painful ulceration, mucosal scleroderma
Gastro-intestinal	Strictures, abnormal gut motility, weight loss
Liver	Cholestasis, abnormal LFTs
Respiratory	Bronchiolitis obliterans, chronic infections including sinusitis
Musculo-skeletal	Fascitis, osteoporosis
Immune system	Functional asplenia, profound immunosuppression, hypogammaglobulinaemia. Risk of pneumoccal sepsis fungal and pneumocystis infections
Haematopoietic system	Cytopenias, eosinophilia

Chronic GvHD results in significant morbidity and reduced quality of life. The commonest cause of death is infection. Symptomatic treatments are very important to keep patients as well as possible for as long as possible. These include moisturizing and sun-blocking skin preparations, artificial tears and saliva, analgesia, physiotherapy, nutritional support, and infection prophylaxis. In view of the many systems involved, care requires co-ordinated input from several multidisciplinary speciality teams.

Systemic therapy usually includes immunosuppression with cyclosporin and steroids, aiming to control disease activity, then to gradually wean treatment. This usually takes 6–9 months. If disease is not controlled, other potentially useful agents include azathioprine, thalidomide, photopheresis, PUVA, mycophenolate mofetil, and tacrolimus. Infection prophylaxis during therapy is important.

Other organ toxicities

Chemotherapy and radiotherapy can have delayed effects. Cataract formation results from TBI and is exacerbated by prolonged steroid treatment of GvHD. Radiotherapy, in particular in children, can cause leucoencephalopathy and neurocognitive problems. Pneumonitis and/or fibrosis due to conditioning or infection such as CMV may occur late, in particular in those receiving continuing immunosupression. Iron overload from repeated red cell transfusion can result in liver impairment but can be treated with venesection.

Infertility and endocrine dysfunction

The majority of allogeneic transplant recipients will be rendered infertile after the procedure, although there have been a few rare cases of conception after a transplant.[6] Alkylating agents and TBI result in gonadal failure, however the effect of recent combination regimens is not yet clear. In women, the risk of premature ovarian failure increases with age and, even if pregnancy is achieved, there is an increased risk of spontaneous abortion and pre-term labour. Adequate hormone replacement post-transplant will help reduce troublesome menopausal symptoms and reduce the risk of osteporosis. Restoration of fertility in men may be achieved by semen storage prior to high-dose therapy. Women may be offered embryo cryopreservation but this requires a partner and time to stimulate ovulation. Egg donation may become available in the future. Other options include adoption.

Endocrine status, including thyroid function, should be checked regularly post-transplant. Hypothyroidism can occur early or late after transplant and should be treated with thyroxine replacement. In children, growth and development should be monitored in specialist clinics.

Relapse

Relapse is a significant cause of treatment failure. The risk of relapse depends upon the disease itself, the status at the time of transplant, and the type of transplant. Patients relapsing after allogeneic transplant may be eligible for donor lymphocyte infusions in an attempt to induce a graft versus disease effect. In those (the majority) in whom cure is no longer an option, all supportive services should be deployed.

Psychological morbidity

Psychological morbidity is seen regularly after transplantation. Indeed, many recipients report symptoms of psychological distress 2–5 years later.[7–9] Presenting symptoms can include low self-esteem, low personal satisfaction with life, and depression.

Secondary malignancy

Secondary malignancy is a recognized consequence of transplantation. Post-transplant lymphoproliferative disorders occur in patients with profound T-cell dysfunction in the presence of EB virus (e.g. T-cell depleted grafts in congenital immune dysfunction). They arise in the first 3–5 months after transplant in <1% of allogeneic transplants.

Secondary myelodysplastic syndromes (MDS) and acute leukaemias have a cumulative incidence of 4% at 5 years, with onset between 3 and 8 years after transplant. Solid organ tumours are also increased and develop later than MDS/acute leukaemia. A recent review suggested an eight-fold increase over expected incidence in those surviving 10 years post-allogeneic transplant. This includes melanoma, oral cavity cancers, liver, CNS, thyroid, and bone.[10] Although the overall incidence is low, longer observation is required to fully assess risks and thus tailor transplant strategies.

Conclusion

Stem cell transplantation involves intensive procedures, which result in mortality and considerable morbidity both at the time of transplant and for years after the procedure. Care of these patients includes specialist multidisciplinary teams supporting the patients at all stages before, during, and after transplant.

References

1 Beyer, J., Schwella, N., Zingsem, J. et al. (1995) Hematopoietic rescue after high-dose chemotherapy using autologous peripheral-blood progenitor cells or bone marrow: a randomized comparison. J Clin Oncol, 13 (6), 1328–35.

2 Marr, K. A., Carter, R. A., Crippa, F. *et al.* (2002) Epidemiology and outcome of mould infections in hematopoietic stem cell transplant recipients. *Clin Infect Dis*, **34**, 909–17.

3 Quabeck, K. (1994) The lung as a critical organ in marrow transplantation. *Bone Marrow Trans*, **14** (suppl. 4), S18–S28.

4 Bearman, S. I., Lee, J. L., Baron, A. E. *et al.* (1997) Treatment of hepatic venocclusive disease with recombinant human tissue plasminogen activator and heparin in 42 marrow transplant patients. *Blood*, **89**, 1501–6.

5 Shulman, H., Sullivan, K. M., Weiden, P. L. *et al.* (1980) Chronic graft versus host disease in man: a clinicopathologic study of 20 long term Seattle patients. *Am J Med*, **69**, 204–17.

6 Apperley, J. F., Rio, B., Ljungman, P. *et al.* (1997) For the Late Effects Working Party of the European Group for Blood and Marrow Transplantation. Outcome of conceptions in male and female patients previously treated by transplantation. *Bone Marrow Transplant*, **19** (suppl. 1), A836.

7 Wolcott, D. L., Wellisch, D. K., Fawzy, I. F. *et al.* (1986) Adaption of adult bone marrow transplant recipient long-term survivors. *Transplantation*, **41**, 478–84.

8 Lesko, L. M. (1994) Bone marrow transplantation: support of the patient and his/her family. *Supp Care Cancer*, **2**, 35–49.

9 Molassiotis, A. (1996) Late psychosocial effects of conditioning for BMT. *Br J Nursing*, **5** (21), 1296–302.

10 Deeg, H. J. and Socie, G. (1998) Malignancies after haematopoietic stem cell transplantation: many questions, some answers. *Blood*, **91**, 1833–44.

Chapter 6

Palliative care for patients undergoing intensive chemotherapy

Paul Perkins and Susan Closs

Introduction

Many patients with haemato-oncological disease receive aggressive chemotherapy with the aim of cure. These regimens cause adverse effects that can be a considerable burden for the patient, and a management challenge for the clinician. They may also lead to delay or cessation of treatment.

In contrast to some other malignancies, there can be a rapid transition for the patient from feeling well to undergoing intensive treatment. This can have a dramatic psychological effect and there may not be time for them to be adequately prepared for what they have to face.

If cured, the patient can be left with long-term sequelae; if treatment fails, the change to terminal care can be sudden and traumatic; and, because of its radical nature, some will die as a result of treatment.

The disease and its treatment will have a significant impact on every aspect of the patient's life. Both will also have wide-ranging effects on the family. An integrated approach from a flexible palliative care multidisciplinary team working with, and alongside, the haematology team is essential to support both patient and family. The involvement of the palliative care team can be helpful from the time of diagnosis.

Working with potentially curable diseases is relatively new for palliative care services, which have their origin in hospices and community teams whose definition of service states that active treatment has ceased. In cancer (or solid tumours) patients may not respond and there is a well-defined point at which curative therapy is withdrawn and the team changes to a palliative approach. In young haematology patients the withdrawal of aggressive treatment happens late in the course of the disease. For the doctor it will mean that they must be particularly mindful of the risk–benefit of all therapy. For everyone in the team it means maintaining a delicate balance because the patient and family are not facing death, at least consciously, when undergoing intensive treatment, even when the prognosis is statistically poor.

Evidence

Intensive chemotherapy is an area of active research. There has been much work in the form of well co-ordinated, randomized, multicentre, trials—investigating the best modes of treatment and management of side-effects. There is less work looking at supportive therapy and rehabilitation.

Psychosocial concerns

Points to remember:

1. Cancer is a diagnosis with wide-ranging effects on the patient and family. Even the words cancer and leukaemia are dreaded, and the diagnosis alone will alter patients' views of their world drastically.

2. Diagnosis is soon followed by treatment with its own burdens. Time spent having, and recovering after, treatment means that patients will not be able to work or care for others for a considerable time. Roles may have to be reversed with parents being cared for by children.

3. Patients are often surprised by the various symptoms, including fatigue, that treatment brings. These can be particularly difficult to bear if they had not been feeling unwell prior to chemotherapy. Frequently diagnosis is a chance finding on investigation of relatively minor symptoms in a previously fit person.

4. A feeling of isolation is common and this may be pronounced if treatment demands reverse barrier nursing in single accommodation or isolation in laminar-flow rooms. They can also miss out on the support that cancer patients find from talking to each other on open wards.

5. The course of disease can be one of remission followed by relapse, providing its own emotional stress. For patients in remission, the prospect of recurrence hangs over them.

6. There can be long-term effects from intensive treatment. Fatigue, breathlessness, skin disease, steroid-induced myopathy, and chemotherapy-induced neuropathy are among some of the sequelae, which can be a burden to patients who are cured.

7. Self-image is commonly affected. Some feel that their own body is turning against itself but there are often more visible changes. Hair loss can be traumatic; choosing an appropriate wig may be helpful before treatment

begins. A Hickman line is a constant reminder of disease, and skin graft versus host disease (GvHD) can alter appearance.

8. A rapid transition from curative to palliative treatment can be bewildering for patient and family. With many cancers there is often weeks, months, or even years between the institution of palliative treatment and death. In haematology this time may be very short, so the patient is not able to come to terms with the future. This may also mean that bereavement is more likely to be pathological for relatives. This transition is covered in more detail in Chapter 10.

9. Disease will put financial pressure on the patient and family, particularly if the patient with disease is the breadwinner. It is vital that families are advised about the help they can get both from the state and charities.

10. A significant proportion of patients with leukaemia are teenagers or young adults. There are often enormous strains on family relationships as parents and their young adult children are torn between the normal process of separating from each other and yet feeling very protective of each other and needing support. Siblings may feel jealous of attention given to the 'sick child'; parental relationships will be affected by tiredness, worry, and even feelings of guilt.

Depression

Patients with malignant disease can become depressed—the research literature suggests that clinical depression is under diagnosed in most cancer centres. As well as affecting the quality of life of both the patient and their family, depression (and anxiety) can affect the success of medical treatments such as bone marrow transplant. The tiredness, sleep disturbance, and loss of appetite that can be part of cancer can mimic the biological symptoms of depression. Therefore symptoms such as anhedonia and guilty ruminations become more important in making the diagnosis. Depression measures such as the hospital anxiety and depression scale, which focus on psychological rather than physical symptoms, may be particularly useful in screening for this condition. There is a spectrum of low mood from adjustment reaction to depression, and the diagnosis can be difficult.

In addition, some of the drug therapy used in the treatment of haematological malignancies can cause psychological symptoms: for example, patients taking high doses of corticosteroids can become agitated or depressed, and the immunosuppressant drug tacrolimus has been associated with dysphoria. Every team should have the input of a psychologist or psychiatrist, who has an interest in and knowledge of psycho-oncology, in order to provide the best care to these patients and their families.

It is desirable to prepare people psychologically to undergo intensive treatment regimens that involve prolonged hospital stays with much-reduced social contact and support. This should be possible, although it is rare, for 'planned' events such as transplants but is more difficult for intensive treatment for acute leukaemia, which frequently commences on the day of diagnosis.

For more information see Chapters 8 and 10.

Nausea and vomiting

The problem

Between 70 and 80% of chemotherapy patients experience nausea and vomiting. While newer anti-emetics, such as selective 5-HT_3 receptor antagonists, have revolutionized the care of cancer patients, emesis is still a major problem[1] and it can be very disabling and distressing. About one-third of patients will also be troubled by anticipatory nausea. Most nausea and vomiting in this setting will be related to chemotherapy or radiotherapy, but it is vital to exclude other aetiologies. It is always important to establish if the patient has nausea or vomiting or both together.

Aetiology

There are numerous possible causes of nausea and vomiting, including:

(1) chemotherapy;

(2) gastric stasis—this can be associated with paraneoplastic autonomic neuropathy; upper abdominal lymphadenopathy; constipation; or it may be drug-induced, e.g. opioids, tricyclic antidepressants;

(3) gastritis—from non-steroidal anti-inflammatory drugs;

(4) biochemical changes—hypercalcaemia, uraemia;

(5) raised intracranial pressure, which affects the vomiting centre;

(6) pharyngeal stimulation caused by oral candidiasis;

(7) pain;

(8) anxiety;

(9) anticipatory or conditioned vomiting—from previous chemotherapy or past experience predating the treatment for cancer, but reawakened by it, e.g. patients who have experienced hyperemesis gravidarum, severe vomiting after surgery, or serious travel sickness may be more likely to experience nausea and vomiting with chemotherapy;

(10) coincidental due to co-existing conditions, e.g. vestibular disease, autonomic neuropathy secondary to diabetes mellitus.

Assessment

A thorough assessment is essential and a good history is always the starting point. Open questions allow the patient to talk and air his or her chief concerns.

History

There are clues in the history that will help elicit the possible cause(s):

(1) the timing of the symptom in relation to chemotherapy or drugs;

(2) patients with biochemical causes often feel nauseated, while those with gastric stasis may not feel very sick;

(3) pattern of vomiting—gastric stasis causes vomiting of sudden onset that relieves nausea, while biochemical causes can lead the patient to have several small vomits throughout the day;

(4) other symptoms—nausea may be related to pain and/or anxiety, and there may be headaches suggestive of raised intracranial pressure;

(5) other medical problems will be elicited by a good history.

Examination

This should be thorough and systematic. Do not forget to examine the mouth thoroughly, as oral candidiasis may give a clue to the cause. A distended or painful abdomen will also be significant, and the character or absence of bowel sounds is also important. Remember that some chemotherapy agents and other drug treatments can cause an ileus.

Rectal examination should be considered but never used in neutropenic patients at risk of abscess or sepsis.

Investigations

Important basic investigations include renal and liver function tests, and serum corrected calcium. Plain films of the abdomen can be helpful. Cranial computed axial tomography (CT) may be indicated if raised intracranial pressure is suspected and advanced imaging techniques are needed to assess the abdomen and pelvis, as disease progression may cause bowel obstruction particularly in NHL. Nausea and vomiting may be caused by neutropenic enterocolitis in patients with acute leukaemia (see Chapter 3 for more details).

Management—drug treatment

Pharmacotherapy is the mainstay of treatment, although general palliative measures such as good communication, explanation of the possible causes, and honest reassurance should be used for all patients. The family should be sought out and kept informed of what is happening—the patient may feel too exhausted to keep them up to date. Whilst waiting for the results of investigations, active treatment of the symptom(s) is essential—this includes frequent reassessment of the effectiveness of any drugs or other measures used.

Chemotherapy—related nausea

Most studies of anti-emetics have been conducted on patients receiving cisplatin chemotherapy, and although cisplatin is not commonly used in haematological malignancies, it is thought that data can be extrapolated to nausea and vomiting caused by other agents.

A schematic representation of the pathways involved in the genesis of nausea and vomiting is shown in Fig. 6.1 and more information is outlined in Chapter 8.

The choice of anti-emetic is affected by a number of factors:

(1) the emetogenicity of the chemotherapy;

(2) the age of the patient (young and old seem to be more vulnerable to extra-pyramidal side-effects from metoclopramide, for example);

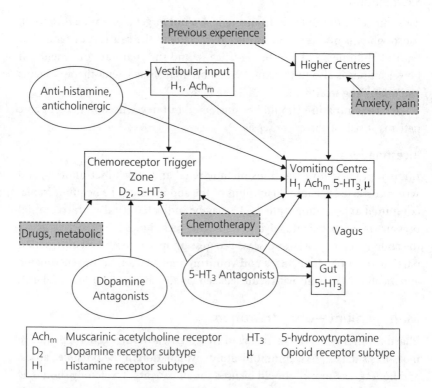

Ach_m	Muscarinic acetylcholine receptor	HT_3	5-hydroxytryptamine
D_2	Dopamine receptor subtype	μ	Opioid receptor subtype
H_1	Histamine receptor subtype		

Fig. 6.1 Schematic representation of nausea and vomiting pathways.

(3) the degree of sedation the patient will tolerate;

(4) symptoms from previous cycles.

For highly emetogenic chemotherapy, 5-HT$_3$ receptor antagonists and corticosteroids (e.g. dexamethasone) are often used in combination. For less emetogenic chemotherapy, dexamethasone alone or combined with other drugs such as metoclopramide can be used.

Gastric stasis

A prokinetic agent such as metoclopramide will be useful.

Biochemical nausea

A dopamine antagonist such as haloperidol is first-line treatment. It acts at the chemoreceptor trigger zone.

Drugs working at the vomiting centre and higher centres include:

- cyclizine (an anti-cholinergic and anti-histamine)
- lorazepam has a role in the management of anxiety and may help prevent anticipatory nausea.

Other considerations

Route of administration

This is important. For patients who are vomiting, oral anti-emetics will not be absorbed, so parenteral administration by intravenous or continuous subcutaneous infusion should be considered. It is important to prescribe 'as needed' anti-emetics in addition to the infusion. Be careful not to write up drugs simultaneously that have opposing modes of action, such as cyclizine and metoclopramide.

Treating the cause

Once anti-emetic treatment has been instituted, consideration should be given to reversing the possible underlying cause. If emesis is secondary to hypercalcaemia, for example, treatment with intravenous fluids and bisphophshonates will often alleviate symptoms. If the nausea is drug-induced it may be possible to alter the patient's medication.

Surgical problems

Although unusual, the patient may have a surgical abdomen. Vomiting may be caused by intussusception secondary to small bowel lymphoma, for example. The extent of disease and prognosis need to be taken into account but it might be appropriate to involve the surgical team in the patient's care.

Non-drug treatment

There is evidence that behavioural interventions can play a role in the treatment of nausea and vomiting. These techniques may be particularly useful in anticipatory emesis, as this is thought to occur because of classical Pavlovian conditioning. The following approaches have produced some success but do depend on local expertise:

1. Hypnosis.
2. Progressive muscle relaxation. This is a technique where patients tense and relax different muscle groups. It seems that it can help reduce negative affect and nausea and vomiting.
3. Distraction techniques. These have been used and one study demonstrated that video games can reduce emesis in children.
4. Guided imagery. This involves patients imagining themselves in alternative, relaxing locations. One study combined guided imagery with music therapy and showed a decreased duration of nausea.
5. Systematic desensitization may also help anticipatory nausea.

The role of acupuncture

Acupuncture has been advocated for many conditions and a recent meta-analysis examined its role and showed that it can help nausea and vomiting.[2] It should be avoided in patients who are thrombocytopenic or neutropenic, but acupressure can be used instead.

Mucositis

The problem

Mucositis is a difficult symptom. Estimates vary but it occurs in approximately 50% of patients who have systemic chemotherapy and is almost invariable in patients receiving intensive regimens. None of the current approaches to prevention and symptom control is completely successful. In addition to outlining current practice, recent advances and other developing approaches are considered below. A fuller account will be found in Chapter 7.

Mucositis may be more common in patients with haematological malignancies, than in those with solid tumours for the following reasons:

- higher doses of chemotherapy are used
- the patients are younger—youth is thought to increase susceptibility because of the increased rate of cell turnover.

Assessment

For mucositis, the assessment of the patient should begin ideally before chemotherapy starts, so that sources of infection or irritation can be identified and corrected, if possible. The assistance of a dentist or dental hygienist in this pretreatment phase is invaluable, although because of the need to start treatment rapidly it is not always possible to obtain it.

Once chemotherapy has begun, the patient may complain of oral pain, dry mouth, dysphagia, and taste disturbance. Daily, careful examination of the oral cavity is vital.

There are several different rating scales for mucositis and, although it seems there can be inter-observer variability between scores, they can be helpful as part of assessment.

Management—non-drug treatment

Treatment of caries and periodontal disease, and correction of sources of irritation such as false teeth, is needed before chemotherapy. This may reduce the frequency of mucositis. It is not always possible, especially when therapy begins abruptly.

Oral hygiene is important during therapy and daily brushing with a soft toothbrush, flossing, and rinsing with saline and dilute sodium bicarbonate, can all have a role. During an episode of mucositis itself, toothbrushing and flossing are often avoided, as even minor trauma may lead to bleeding or bacteraemia—especially if there is concomitant thrombocytopenia or neutropenia. Swab sticks soaked in sodium bicarbonate can be used instead. Lip lubrication and the use of saliva substitutes aid comfort. For more information on mouth care see Chapter 7.

There is conflicting evidence in the literature, and a great variety of mouth-care regimens are used across the world. Mucositis should be anticipated in patients receiving intensive treatment and therefore excellent care should be instigated from the beginning to reduce the severity of the condition. A summary of what is known about the management of mucositis is outlined below.

Management of mucositis

This should always include:

1. Assessment and preparation of the oral cavity before or early in treatment.
2. Early detection of problems: daily examination and direct questioning of the patient about symptoms such as pain, dryness, and taste disturbance is vital.
3. Good mouth care: this includes excellent cleaning of teeth and gums.

4. Active treatment of pain. Strong opioids are indicated for severe pain. If it becomes impossible to take oral medication, then the intravenous or subcutaneous routes can be used. Patient controlled analgesia (PCA) seems to be most effective and well-tolerated, and results in a lower opioid dose than continuous infusion. Morphine or diamorphine should be opioids of first choice.

5. Early treatment of infections such as candidiasis and herpes simplex.

6. Good general care, e.g. the maintenance of nutrition and hydration.

Recent advances and possible research developments in drug treatment

A recent Cochrane review examined the treatments for oral mucositis.[3] It suggested that there is weak evidence to support the use of allopurinol and vitamin E mouthwashes.

There are three main avenues of investigation for the prevention or treatment of mucositis:

1. To reduce infection, inflammation and pain from the mucositis:
   a. Chlorhexidine is an antiseptic mouthwash and early studies showed that it might be able to prevent mucositis. More recent randomized studies revealed that it has little impact and may even *increase* pain.
   b. Sucralfate is used to treat gastro-intestinal ulceration and it is thought to form a protective layer over ulcers. For mucositis, the literature is conflicting and it appears to have a limited role.
   c. Benzydamine is a topical non-steroidal with analgesic, anaesthetic, anti-inflammatory, and antimicrobial properties. While some studies have shown it provides analgesia, others disagree.
   d. Other topical agents, such as local anaesthetics and capsaicin, have been used with little evidence to support them.

2. To decrease the exposure of the mucosa to the chemotherapy:
   a. Allopurinol has been investigated for mucositis induced by 5-fluorouracil (5-FU), as it is known to inhibit an enzyme involved in its metabolism. As 5-FU is not used in haemato-oncology, it is unlikely that it will have a role in mucositis in this setting.
   b. Etoposide is excreted in the saliva. It was hoped that the anticholinergic, propantheline bromide, might decrease salivation and reduce mucositis. The results of a small trial have been encouraging.

c. The possibility that topical folinic acid could reduce the impact of systemic methotrexate was suggested but the results of a non-randomized study were not encouraging.

d. Chronotherapy: DNA synthesis seems to decrease in oral mucosa between the hours of midnight and 4 a.m. Chemotherapy can, therefore, have a differential effect depending on its timing.

e. Cryotherapy: this involves placing crushed ice in the mouth to cause vasoconstriction, decreasing the delivery of chemotherapeutic agents. Several trials have shown benefits with 5-FU, but it may also help with toxicity from melphalan.

3. To alter mucosal proliferation:

a. Corticosteroids may help by reducing prostaglandin and leukotriene production. A pilot study in radiation-induced mucositis showed that this might become an option in the future.

b. The vitamin A derivatives, betacarotene and tretinoin, as well as the prostaglandins, dinprostone and misoprostol, have been tried in small studies with varying success.

c. A randomized trial showed no benefit of oral glutamine in the prevention of 5-FU-induced mucositis.

d. Vitamin E seems to stabilize cell membranes, perhaps as an antioxidant, and it led to resolution of mucositis in the treatment group in a small randomized controlled trial.

Haematopoietic growth factors (HGFs) are naturally occurring cytokines that have differential effects on different types of blood cell. Granulocyte colony stimulating factor (G-CSF) and granulocyte macrophage colony stimulating factor (GM-CSF) may be helpful in the prevention and treatment of mucositis. Studies have shown that these factors seem to protect the oral mucosa. This may be because of their effect on neutrophils, while some think they may stimulate the mucosa directly. Other cytokines are undergoing investigation.

Rehabilitation and palliative care

There are many ways in which intensive treatment can have a detrimental impact on a patient's physical ability to function:

1. Patients are in bed for prolonged periods. This can cause changes in cardiovascular physiology. Fluid shifts from the legs to the thorax, and there is a diuresis. This leads to postural hypotension and even left ventricular atrophy if bed-rest is prolonged. Red cell volume remains constant, so

there is elevated blood viscosity leading to increased risk of thrombo-embolic disease. Patients will require a graded return to normal activity and need to be helped to remain active.

2. In between admissions to hospital, patients may feel mentally and physically fatigued and avoid exercise—this compounds the loss of muscle mass that occurs with prolonged bed rest or lack of exercise associated with in-patient treatment. About 1% of muscle strength is lost per day of bed-rest. Anaemia will compound fatigue.

3. Some chemotherapeutic agents (e.g. vincristine) can cause polyneuropathy. This will limit mobility further. If it is painful, analgesics will be needed. If it causes weakness, orthoses can help function so encouraging activity.

4. Steroids cause proximal myopathy leading to weakness, particularly on movements such as rising from a chair or brushing the hair.

5. Patients need to be encouraged to maintain mobility as much as possible during treatment. If frail, assisted or passive movements can help. Rehabilitation physicians, occupational therapists (OTs), and physiotherapists can all help patients to maintain their independence as much as possible.

6. Even after treatment the patient may have a significantly reduced functional capacity[4] and an accurate assessment of their physical abilities is the first step. If a rehabilitation physician is involved he/she will measure the patient's abilities and problems before treatment begins. A management plan will be agreed with the patient and standard outcome measures used to quantify improvements.

7. Exercise can have a positive effect on a patient's morale. There is evidence that it improves functional capacity in many other medical conditions— the patient will need encouragement to maintain and develop an exercise programme, as they are likely to feel worse when they first start exerting themselves.

Breathlessness

This is a late complication of intensive treatment—for example, it may be associated with lung damage following chemotherapy, with GvHD, or treatment-related cardiac failure. Patients are often young and want to follow careers, look after their families, and keep up socially with their friends. Palliative care physicians will be involved in the long-term when treatment to reverse the underlying cause has been exhausted.

A positive attitude from the physician will help the patient to persist with active symptom control—frequently patients will feel nihilistic by the time they see the palliative care physician. They will have endured very demanding treatment followed by disappointment at its partial failure and their disablement. Treatment programmes should be multidisciplinary and planned for each individual depending on their diagnosis and the degree of activity they can undertake when first seen.

Simple measures include:

1. All patients should be encouraged to be as active as possible—deconditioning will only exacerbate their breathlessness.

2. Patients and their families need to understand that breathlessness is not of itself dangerous, although unpleasant—breathlessness resulting from the late complications of intensive treatment is not likely to cause the patients to die gasping for breath, and it is less likely to be progressive.

3. Episodes of breathlessness are often precipitated by anxiety—exploring the patient's interpretation of the symptom and their fears associated with it may enable a clinician to help the patient to alter their cognitions about the symptom and allay their anxiety. Psychologists, physiotherapists or clinical nurse specialists may be particularly skilled at this.

4. Teaching the patient to cool their face with a fan in the distribution of the 2nd and 3rd branches of the 5th cranial nerve has been shown to reduce breathlessness. A hand-held fan is a portable convenient way of reducing the severity of the symptom.

5. Breathing and relaxation exercises may be very helpful and can be quickly taught on the ward or in out-patients.

Pharmacological treatments

Opioids and benzodiazepines will not usually be appropriate for those patients who are frequently breathless on exertion only.

Ambulatory oxygen, i.e. the use of oxygen during the activities of daily living, may be very helpful. The patient should undergo a formal exercise test with and without oxygen. Oxygen should be prescribed if the patient is symptomatically better on oxygen, or if they are able to increase their exercise capacity by 10% using oxygen, or if they desaturate below 90% on exercise whilst breathing air. Breathlessness should be assessed using standardized tools such as the visual analogue scale or Borg scale.

Diarrhoea

This can be associated with intensive chemotherapy, or may be caused by a complication of the underlying disease and is also a manifestation of GvHD. The diagnosis is essential to finding a correct treatment. There are some specific regimens to treat the acute diarrhoea associated with particular chemotherapy agents: for example, using regular frequent loperamide or codeine phosphate—details of these are supplied by the pharmaceutical company. If the diarrhoea is not controlled, drugs that reduce the volume of intestinal secretions, such as hyoscine butylbromide and octreotide, alone or in combination, may be used. These are usually given as a continuous subcutaneous infusion. Constant review of the drug regimen is important and attention should be paid to the details of the general aspects of the patient's condition such as nutrition and hydration. The palliative care physician will be working in an advisory capacity in these circumstances.

Dry skin

This is a common problem in patients—the skin must be kept as moist and lubricated as possible, preferably with ointments free of preservatives and perfumes.

Sunburn must be avoided, as it will exacerbate the condition. Patients should observe sensible precautions, such as avoiding direct sun between 11 a.m. and 3 p.m., and wearing hats and suitable clothing. They should also use a high protection sun-block (factor 25) that is effective against UVA and B.

The sweat glands are sometimes affected and patients need to take care to avoid overheating.

Dry eyes will benefit from artificial tears.

References

1 Abraham, J. L. (2000). Pain management and antiemetic therapy in haematologic disorders. In *Hematology: Basic principles and practice* (ed. R. Hoffman, E. J. Benz, S. J. Shattil *et al.*), pp. 1522–34. Churchill Livingstone, New York.
2 Vickers, A. J. (1996). Can acupuncture have specific effects on health? A systematic review of acupuncture antiemesis trials. *J R Soc Med*, **89**, 303–11.
3 Worthington, H. V., Clarkson, J. E., and Eden, O. B. (2002). Interventions for treating oral mucositis for patients with cancer receiving treatment (Cochrane review). The Cochrane Library, Issue 1, Oxford, Update Software.
4 Gillis, T. A. and Donovan, E. S. (2001). Rehabilitation following bone marrow transplant. *Cancer*, **19**, 998–1007.

Chapter 7

Mouth care for haematology patients

Ilora Finley, Pia Amsler, and
Rosemary Wade

Introduction

Disease or treatment-related mouth problems, particularly those associated with chemotherapy or radiotherapy and with other types of immunosuppression, are a common cause of severe pain in haematology patients. Oral problems affect the patient's ability to communicate and to eat, impeding social interaction, as well as distorting taste and altering breathing patterns. In addition, the impaired efficacy of the mucosal barrier and reduced saliva production increases the risk of local and systemic infection, and can potentially require chemotherapy regimen dose reductions, treatment schedule delays, or modifications of drug combinations.

This chapter deals with the causes of oral problems in haematological patients, the pathogenesis of chemotherapy and radiotherapy induced mucositis, the incidence and assessment of oral mucositis, and its prevention and treatment.

The diagnosis, assessment and management of disease-related and treatment-related mouth problems are commonly left to trained nursing staff. As a consequence, most published guidance on the practical aspects of mouth care in oncology and haematology patients is found in the nursing literature. Oral assessment and treatment often follows empirical algorithms, not always taking the patients' individual needs into account. Furthermore, evidence-based research on treatment regimens is unfortunately scarce.

Oral mucositis can severely reduce a patient's quality of life and even their ability to continue with chemo- and radiotherapy. Therefore all clinicians need to be aware of the different components of appropriate mouth care.

For this chapter we are defining:

- *stomatitis* as general inflammation of the oral cavity with multiple aetiologies

- *mucositis* as inflammation of mucous membranes anywhere in the gastro-intestinal tract.

Sources of evidence

There is little scientific evidence on which mouth care can be based. For this chapter, we have reviewed the literature for available evidence. We drew on the Cochrane reviews on the subject and standard textbooks in oncology, haematology, and palliative care, including the *Oxford Textbook of Palliative Medicine*, and undertook a comprehensive Medline review, as well as searching the Internet (references with internet sites). Key references are given at the end of this chapter.

Incidence

Chemotherapy induced oral mucositis is almost inevitable in patients undergoing myeloablative chemotherapy or radiotherapy preceding bone marrow transplantation (BMT). Marked mucositis is less common in those receiving standard curative or palliative chemotherapy regimens.

The extent of mucosal damage is usually related to the dose of the chemotherapeutic agent. Certain schedules carry a higher risk of mucosal injury than others. These include myoablation prior to bone marrow transplantation, high-dose induction therapies, and combinations of chemo- and radiotherapy given concurrently. However, the same treatment regimen can cause mild mucosal injury in some and severe mucositis in others, which suggests there are confounding disease-related, environmental and genetic factors.

The incidence of chemotherapy and radiotherapy induced oral mucosal injury reported from various groups of patients is as follows:

- in patients with solid cancers receiving:
  - adjuvant chemotherapy: 10–15%
  - curative chemotherapy: ca. 40%
- in patients with head and neck cancer, receiving radiotherapy involving the oral cavity: 100%
- in patients with haematological disorders:
  - non-Hodgkin's lymphoma: 30–40%
  - leukaemia: 60–70%
  - receiving a BMT: 70–80%.

Certain groups, such as younger patients and women, are particularly at risk of chemotherapy induced mucositis. Other important risk factors include the patient's nutritional status; pre-existing poor dental hygiene, and pre-existing xerostomia.

Pathogenesis and clinical course of mucositis

Although the oral cavity and oropharynx are clinically most often affected, the underlying pathology extends to all other intestinal mucosal surfaces and symptoms such as dysphagia, dyspepsia, and diarrhoea may occur due to involvement of the oesophagus, stomach, or intestine.

Chemotherapy induced mucositis

Different tissues have different rates of turnover, which has important implications for healing rates. The damage from chemotherapy due to rapidly replicating non-keratinized squamous epithelial surfaces is much greater than to keratinized surfaces.

Cytotoxic agents may act as *initiators, promoters* or *effectors* of mucosal damage. There are several points in the cell cycle that are targeted by chemotherapeutic agents, resulting in cell damage or death.

These cellular mechanisms include:

1. Direct cytotoxicity against proliferating stem cells in the basal epithelium.
2. Indirect cytotoxicity through the epithelium's inability to contain minor oral infection or limit the effect of local trauma during the period of myelosuppression.
3. Tissue injury activation of pro-inflammatory cytokines, e.g. interleukin (IL)-1, IL-6, tumour necrosis factor alpha (TNF-α), interferon gamma (IFN-γ) and IL-2.
4. Probable direct and/or indirect suppression of anti-inflammatory cytokines, e.g. circulating IL-1 receptor (IL-1ra), IL-4, IL-10, and IL-11.
5. Some cytokines (TGF-α; IL-1; epidermal growth factor, EGF; platelet-derived growth factor, PDGF) are also thought to be involved in the stimulation or suppression of epithelial cell proliferation and help to maintain tissue homeostasis. Much attention is currently being paid to the role of cytokines and other humoral transmitters in the pathogenesis of chemotherapy induced mucositis and we refer the reader to the relevant articles for a more detailed account.

A summary of the resulting oral complications from chemotherapy is given in Table 7.1.

Gastro-intestinal epithelial cells have a cell turnover rate similar to leukocytes, so the time frame of mucosal damage is correspondingly similar.

Table 7.1 Oral complications of cancer chemotherapy

Direct toxicity:
  Oral mucositis
  Salivary gland dysfunction
  Neurotoxicity
  —Altered taste
  —Gingival and dental hypersensitivity
  Temporo-mandibular joint dysfunction
  Impaired dental development in children

Indirect toxicity:
  Myelosuppression
  —Neutropenia and immunosuppression
  —Anaemia (myoablative, folate and iron deficiency states)
  —Thrombocytopenia
  Infection
  —Viral
  —Fungal
  —Bacterial
  Mucositis of lower gastro-intestinal tract
  Nausea and vomiting

Resolution of oral toxicity, including mucositis and infection, generally coincides with granulocyte recovery although mucosal healing is delayed in some.

Erythematous patches occasionally appear three days after exposure to chemotherapy. Oral pain is nearly always associated with mucositis and frequently starts shortly after the visible onset; it typically resolves 1–3 days before resolution of the oral mucositis. Ulcerative mucositis, seen particularly in patients undergoing bone marrow transplantation, usually begins 7–10 days after the start of cytotoxic treatment.

Anecdotal evidence suggests that patients who experience mucositis with a specific chemotherapy regimen during the first cycle will typically develop comparable mucositis during subsequent courses of that regimen (Table 7.2).

Radiotherapy induced mucosal injury

In haematological malignancy, head and neck radiotherapy is used in total body irradiation and the treatment of cervical lymph nodes. In contrast to chemotherapy, impairment of cell division caused by radiotherapy is anatomically site-specific. It is dependent upon the type of radiation used (i.e. superficial photons and electrons), the total dose administered, the field size, and the fractionation regimen for radiation exposure.

Table 7.2 Chemotherapeutic agents frequently associated with mucositis

- Anthracyclines: doxorubicin, daunorubicin, epirubicin
- Alkylating agents: cyclophosphamide, busulphan, procarbazine
- Taxanes: docetaxel, paclitaxel
- Vinca alkaloids: vinblastine, vincristine, vinorelbine
- Antimetabolites: methotrexate, 5-fluouracil, hydroxyurea, cytosine arabinoside
- Anti-tumour antibiotics: actinomycin D, bleomycin, mitomycin, mithramycin

Table 7.3 Oral complications of radiotherapy involving the oral area

Acute changes	Chronic changes
Oral mucositis	Mucosal fibrosis and atrophy
Infection	Xerostomia
◆ Fungal	Dental caries
◆ Bacterial	Soft tissue necrosis
Salivary gland dysfunction	Osteoradionecrosis
◆ Sialadenitis	Taste dysfunction
◆ Xerostomia	◆ Dysgeusia
◆ Altered taste	◆ Ageusia
	Muscular/cutaneous fibrosis
	Infection
	◆ Fungal
	◆ Bacterial

Tissues treated with ionizing radiation continue to remain vulnerable throughout the life of the patient: they are more easily damaged by subsequent toxic drug or radiation exposures, and normal physiological repair mechanisms are compromised as a result of permanent cellular and structural damage. Anthracyclines and taxanes can produce a radiation recall effect, of unknown mechanism, which can be seen even years later.

Table 7.3 gives the oral changes associated with radiotherapy involving the peri-oral region.

Several processes occur in irradiated tissue at cellular level:

(1) damage to blood vessels leads to end-arteritis obliterans causing hypovascularity, with tissue ischaemia;

(2) reduced proliferation of basal epithelial cells, causes local atrophy;

(3) connective tissue damage leads to increased vascular permeability, tissue oedema and inflammation;

(4) fibroblast injury results in cell loss and altered function, leading to fibrosis after several months;

(5) osteo-radionecrosis is a particular problem with head and neck radiotherapy and requires meticulous dental care prior to radiotherapy.

Radiotherapy-induced oropharyngeal mucositis can occur with a daily administration of 200 cGy, is invariable with dosages above 1000 cGy, and severe mucositis with ulceration is common at doses above 4000 cGy. Some patients, especially those with HIV-AIDS, are particularly vulnerable to the mucositis.

Assessment

History and examination

Patients should be specifically questioned about oral symptoms particularly dryness, pain and altered taste.

Mouth pain

Mouth pain can either be localized to a well-defined area or be of a generalized diffuse nature. Erosive or ulcerative lesions usually cause mild to moderate sharp pain that can be intensified by sour, spicy, or hot foods. Diffuse stomatitis usually causes burning pain and can be associated with altered taste, predominantly of a bitter metallic quality. Words commonly used to describe oral pain are 'tender', 'sore', and 'irritating', and patients may deny pain preferring another term.

Taste disturbance

Taste disturbance can take many forms but many cancer patients describe taste distortion (dysgeusia), general lack of taste perception (hypogeusia), or a metallic/unpleasant taste.

Mucosal alterations frequently occur before the onset of oral pain. Therefore it is of paramount importance to anticipate mucositis and to routinely examine the mouth to initiate appropriate treatment.

Other issues

Not all oral pathology relates to the treatment of cancer. Previously present peridontitis, angular stomatitis, and aphthous ulceration need to be diagnosed and treated before initiation of therapy.

Graft versus host disease (GvHD) is common in patients who have received allogeneic stem cell transplants and is potentially life-threatening. The patient can develop acute (within days) or chronic (within months) injury to the oral tissues. If severe mucositis develops as well as thrombocytopenia, oral bleeding can occur, which can be very difficult to treat.

Healthcare professionals should therefore always pay particular attention to the examination of the mouth, as this detects treatable conditions such as infections and also demonstrates to the patient the importance of their own mouth care. Patients should be actively encouraged to report any changes early.

Examination

Examination of the mouth should take place with any dentures removed using a torch, spatula, and gloves; whenever possible a dental mirror should be used to see the inner aspect of the gums and teeth. A thorough examination includes inspection and palpation of lips, teeth, tongue, and mucous membranes and should be repeated at regular intervals particularly when patients are receiving chemotherapy.

Assessment tools

Systematic assessment of the oral cavity following treatment allows early identification of toxicity and the initiation of oral hygiene measures designed to prevent or decrease further complications. However, there is often no standardized and validated assessment tool used on wards or in the outpatient setting.

An ideal assessment tool should:

- be routinely used by all healthcare professional involved in the patients' care
- be easy and quick to use
- be objective and reproducible with a high inter-observer correlation
- assess the functional dimension of stomatitis (e.g. ability to eat and speak)
- include the patients' own assessment, e.g. of pain
- clearly describe alterations of the lips, tongue, mucous membranes, gingiva, teeth, throat, quality of saliva, and voice.

Simple functional and structural grading systems are available. Most of them are based on two or three clinical parameters such as erythema or ulceration, pain and problems with eating. These are useful because they are easy to carry out and take cognizance of the patient's functional abilities as a measure of severity (an example is given in Table 7.4).

Rating scales to assess the oral cavity can be completed by the patient or by professionals involved in their care. Self-help patient programs are available to

Table 7.4 Examples from WHO oral mucositis grading systems

| Grade | WHO general grading system | Radiation therapy | Oncology group |
		Objective signs	Subjective symptoms
0	No symptoms	No signs	No symptoms
1	Sore mouth, no ulcers	Erythematous sores	Mild soreness, mild dysphagia, solid diet possible
2	Sore mouth with ulcers, but able to eat	Patchy mucositis (<1/2 mucosa)	Moderate pain, moderate dysphagia, soft diet possible
3	Fluids only	Confluent fibrinous mucositis (>1/2 mucosa)	Severe pain, severe dysphagia, liquids only
4	Unable to eat or drink	Haemorrhage and necrosis	Parenteral or enteral support needed

help prevent mucositis; these formally combine didactic information with self-care exercises and nursing support (PRO-SELF©).

Simple numerical rating scales allow patients to quantify symptoms (e.g. oral pain) and enable clinician to rate a clinical finding (e.g. mucositis).

Verbal categorical scales, giving verbal descriptors (e.g. 'sore', 'burning', etc.), are usually used when the nurse or doctor administers the assessment. Verbal scales should not replace exploratory direct questioning and examination of the patient, as the scales only provide a limited assessment.

Newer assessment tools include, for example, the Oral Assessment Guide.[1] This is a clinically orientated evaluation tool that gives three rating scales in each of eight assessment categories. It also assesses the functional impairment caused by mucositis. Other tools include the use of analgesia as a guide of the severity of tissue damage.

The Oral Mucositis Index[2] is a research-orientated tool, which consists of 30 items, divided into anatomic regions of the oral cavity, to specifically assess acute oral mucositis after bone marrow transplantation.

A variety of assessment tools are also available from the National Cancer Institute and sources unrelated to haemato-oncology, e.g. the British Society for Disability and Oral Health, and HIVdent guidelines.

Unfortunately, no single tool has been found to include all the required information in a user-friendly and efficient way. However, complex assessment tools can be simplified and simple descriptive tools can be extended, enabling a unit to adjust an assessment tool to their particular use.

Management

General mouth care for patients undergoing treatment for haematological malignancy

In order to optimize compliance, the patient should understand the reasons why mouth care is important with regard to their disease and treatments.

General recommendations

- Brush with fluoride tooth paste (a small soft tooth brush if easier to use) twice a day.
- Flossing, depending on the individual patient's condition.
- Rinse with water or mouthwash.
- Good denture care.
- Keep lips moist with lip salve.
- See dentist and/or hygienist for teeth and gum care.
- Avoid very hot food and drinks.
- Avoid drinking spirits and smoking.

If the patient is physically unable to brush their own teeth, then this must be done for them. In the past, nurses have preferred not to use brushes but there is established evidence that brushes are more effective than sponges or alternatives at removing plaque. Saline, bicarbonate of soda, or proprietary brand mouthwashes can be used as an adjunct to brushing. If a brush cannot be tolerated due to sensitivity or pain, then sponges on sticks or even a gauze-wrapped finger can be used on the teeth and mucosa. Patients may need general information on diet or to see a dietician in order to optimize their calorific intake without too much sugar.

There is a wide variation in mouth-care protocols for patients who are neutropenic and thrombocytopenic, reflecting the paucity of research in the field. Protocols usually recommend avoiding flossing, and sometimes recommend avoiding brushing. They prefer antiseptics, antifungal mouthwashes, and gels despite their relative ineffectiveness in removing plaque compared to gentle brushing with toothpaste.

Dental assessment

Those patients likely to develop mucositis should be seen by a dental surgeon with knowledge of haemato-oncology, prior to chemotherapy. Carious teeth can be restored and if gingival disease is present, treatment (e.g. chlorhexidine gluconate mouthwashes) can be started prior to chemotherapy. The aim of the assessment is to avoid dental procedures during chemotherapy and to reduce the risk of oral infections. A hygienist may be helpful. Patients with thrombocytopenia may require platelet support prior to certain dental procedures. Close liaison must be maintained between the dentist and the haematology team so that prophylactic antibiotic cover and platelet transfusions may be given where appropriate.

Symptom control

As well as specific treatments, for good palliation patients require symptomatic treatments and general mouth care. Choosing symptom-control measures requires an assessment of the risks and benefits of each treatment.

Dryness

Dry mouth (or xerostomia) can be a chronic condition in these patients, and simple measures are often best. Patients should increase the frequency of oral hygiene up to four hourly, using mouthwashes as mentioned in general mouth care. Frequent drinks, sips of water and ice should be encouraged; humidified air, particularly in the bedroom, may help.

Artificial salivas are often compound preparations based on carboxymethylcellulose, mucin, and salts to moisten and coat the mucosa and tongue. The benefits are often short-lived and some preparations are acid (Glandosane®) and therefore can damage the teeth; they should be avoided in long-term use. If the saliva substitutes are to be used for some time they should contain fluoride (Saliva Orthana®, Luborant®).

Attempts can be made to stimulate saliva production using sugar-free chewing gums, sweets, citrus foods, and sialogues, such as pilocarpine. These only work with intact salivary glands. All medications should be reviewed, stopping those with any anticholinergic action wherever possible, and dehydration avoided.

Coating on tongue/mouth

Frail patients with dry mouths often develop a coated tongue, which feels unpleasant and can reduce taste. The dorsum of the tongue can be cleaned with a brush and chlorhexidine if tolerated, or by sucking pineapple chunks or a quarter effervescent vitamin C tablet. Dentures should be soaked in antiseptic solution and left to dry completely before re-use. A persistently coated tongue may indicate a chronic fungal condition. Hydrogen peroxide, or sodium perborate solution, can be useful for debriding lesions but should only be used for short periods, as it may delay healing. Sodium bicarbonate mouthwash may be an effective alternative.

Angular stomatitis

Angular stomatitis presents as moist or encrusted sores and fissures at the corners of the mouth, usually bilateral. The cause is often multifactorial, including infection, dry lips, nutritional deficiencies, and dentures. In denture wearers infection is almost inevitably fungal, but in the dentate an encrusted lesion is likely to be bacterial or mixed. Palliation will therefore often involve optimization of diet, good mouth care including lip salves, together with treating any infection with topical antifungal and/or antibacterial gels.

Pain

The pain of mouth conditions should be assessed and treated in the same way as pain elsewhere. Patients should be given an explanation of the condition with an expected time course and an explanation of analgesics with regular and as required options. Transient conditions, even when severe, can often be coped with better than chronic ones. The choice of analgesic will depend on whether the mouth pain is local or generalized, and its character and severity.

NSAIDs Benzydamine hydrochloride (Difflam®) is a NSAID with anaesthetic and antimicrobial properties available as an oral rinse or spray. However, soluble paracetamol or any NSAIDs dissolved in warm water can be used as a rinse or swallowed if systemic effects are required. For a local effect, choline salicylate gel (Bonjela®) is useful, but excessive application can itself cause ulceration. Please note that systemic NSAIDs are contra-indicated in thrombocytopenia.

Cytoprotectants Gelatin-based pastes (Orabase®) or mucin-based artificial saliva (Orthana Saliva®) can be applied as a protective coat to areas of ulceration. Carbenoxolone sodium and carmellose gelatin paste relieve discomfort by adhering to ulcer base and are said to promote healing of mild oral lesions. Sucralfate is a cytoprotectant, which is available as a suspension and can be applied topically by rinsing with it; when swallowed it does not reduce gastric acidity.

Local anaesthetics Local anesthetics may give some pain relief but there is a risk of sensitization. Cocaine 2% is a useful local anaesthetic but should be used only as a rinse and not swallowed, due to systemic effects. Proprietary local anaesthetics are available in many forms, as mouth rinses, sprays, gels, or lozenges. Lignocaine 2% is often combined with an antacid (co-magaldrox) or steroid (hydrocortisone 2%) with good effect. Care has to be taken with the timing of application and meals to avoid aspiration, as the oropharynx becomes anaesthetized.

Capsaicin Capsaicin is the active ingredient from chili peppers that produces burning pain. The depolarization block it causes produces late onset numbness and hence pain relief. In theory the pain threshold can be gradually elevated by repeated application of increasing concentrations, as shown by a small case series. It also is mildly sialogue in action.

Antacids Viscous antacids can be used to coat the mouth prior to meals. When antacids are swallowed they may reduce protection against infection from gastric acid, and therefore in patients at risk of systemic infections these preparations may be best used as rinses.

Opioids Morphine can be used topically dissolved in a carrier gel or as oral solution (Oramorph®). When local measures are inadequate or cannot be tolerated, additional systemic analgesia is needed. Systemic analgesics should be chosen according to the WHO analgesic ladder (see Chapter 8).

If a patient's mouth is too sore to take drugs orally, strong opioids may need to be given parenterally or transdermally. As the pain is constant, the analgesics should be given regularly by patient-controlled devices (PCA) or by continuous infusion. Trials have shown opioids to be effective by both these methods, although with PCA the overall dose of opioid used is often lower. Transdermal fentanyl has been shown to be effective, but the time gap until the onset of pain relief with the transdermal formulation allows its use only in prolonged mucositis. However, parenteral fentanyl can be effectively used in patients who are intolerant of diamorphine. Patients on strong opioids usually require laxatives, but this constipating effect of opioids may be of benefit in patients with concomitant diarrhoea from intestinal mucositis.

The 'soreness' of mucositis has similar character to the burning and tingling of neuropathic pain, and amitriptyline was reported as being effective in one trial for some patients. However, its usefulness may be limited due to its anticholinergic properties.

Analgesia should be reviewed regularly for benefits and side-effects. Patients who are depressed will need specific treatment for depression as well as analgesia; strongly anticholinergic drugs should be avoided.

Inability to eat/drink

The mouth conditions severe enough to prevent the patient eating are usually mucositis and infections; diet should be adjusted (soft food at room temperature rather than rough, salty, acidic, or highly spiced food). Local and systemic analgesics should be optimized and given before the patient attempts to eat. Patients may be able to tolerate cold (ice chips) better than warm or vice versa. Nasogastric tubes are very unpleasant for the patient, and are to be avoided in thrombocytopenia. Short periods of starvation are usually tolerated if the nutritional status prior to the treatment was satisfactory. Consideration of parenteral nutrition must take account of the patient's general condition, their nutritional intake over the previous six weeks, and the length of time the mucositis is likely to continue. Parenteral nutrition is often given routinely in patients undergoing bone marrow transplantation. The patient should be encouraged to drink and chew as soon they are able to in order to aid the restoration of a healthy mouth.

Taste disturbance

Disturbance of taste can be a distressing symptom and whether treatment- or disease-related, can continue throughout the illness. This is particularly distressing when combined with a poor appetite.

Patients find it helpful to know this is not unusual; there is written advice available for patients and families regarding diet and foods to try. A dietician can often help. The disturbance can take the form of general decrease or loss of the sense of taste, changes in food preferences, or a specific unpleasant or metallic taste. Xerostomia contributes to poor taste (see above). For those patients with metallic taste, haloperidol (0.5–1.5 mg at night) can be helpful. In patients who have been ill for some time, nutritional deficiencies, particularly trace elements, should be considered. Patients may benefit from a course of zinc, although the evidence is conflicting.

Prevention and treatment of specific mouth conditions

Xerostomia—dry mouth

Certain diseases and treatments may make xerostomia inevitable, but, if anticipated, additional mouth care can be encouraged. It may seem obvious but patients who are not eating and drinking will get xerostomia. This includes patients with nausea, little appetite, those on restricted food and fluids, 'nil by mouth', or with enteral or parenteral feeding. Mastication is important for saliva production and mouth health. Mouth breathing or oxygen therapy can add to a dry mouth and humidification of the room or oxygen may prevent this. Medications causing xerostomia should be avoided if possible. Patients particularly at risk are those who are immunosuppressed—other risk factors include physical disability and diabetes mellitus.

Sialogues Pilocarpine (tablets or oral drops) stimulates secretion from exocrine glands, particularly of the mucin-rich minor saliva glands that protect the mucosa from trauma and dryness. Pilocarpine has been shown to be beneficial in patients receiving chemotherapy, as well as the terminally ill. In a study of patients with dry mouth from cancer, up to 75% reported benefit but 25% had to stop pilocarpine due to adverse effects, particularly sweating, headache, and dizziness.

Saliva-stimulating tablets contain fruit acids and should be pH buffered to avoid teeth sensitivity and caries.

Stomatitis

General inflammation and ulceration of the mouth has many causes. Prevention and treatment will depend on the cause and aims to minimize secondary infection. Causes and associated treatments include:

(1) all cases—optimize mouth hygiene;

(2) physical trauma, e.g. from ill-fitting dentures or uneven teeth requires dental advice;

(3) chemical trauma, e.g. sensitization to mouthwashes and alcohol;

(4) single aphthous ulcers—topical steroids (hydrocortisone lozenges or triamcinolone 0.1% paste) can be placed on the ulcer to suppress the local immune response—self-limiting condition;

(5) general inflammation—antiseptic mouthwash (e.g. chlorhexidine 0.2% aqueous) is used, preparations containing alcohol should be avoided as these can cause stinging, steroid rinses can also be helpful but increase the risk of candidiasis;

(6) nutrition—with the rapid mucosal cell turnover the oral cavity is a sensitive indicator of adequate nutritional status (see Table 7.5);

(7) infections (see below);

(8) chemotherapy (see below).

Prevention of chemotherapy induced mucositis For the prevention of mucositis, general measures include optimizing mouth hygiene and avoiding a dry mouth and lips. Mouth care should be encouraged after each meal and at night with atraumatic cleansing combined with antiseptic rinses.

Interventions for preventing oral mucositis in patients with cancer are the subject of a Cochrane review. No prophylactic agents (including

Table 7.5 Oral features associated with nutritional deficiency and excess

Clinical feature	Nutritional deficiency	Nutritional excess
Scurvy-red swollen gingiva	Vitamin C	
Gingival friability	Vitamins C, B_{12}, Folic acid, copper	
Peridontal destruction	Vitamin C	
Angular stomatitis	Vitamins B group, folic acid, iron	
Oral stomatitis	Vitamins B group, C, folic acid	
Xerostomia	Vitamin A	
Increased risk of bleeding	Vitamin K, calcium	
Incomplete mineralization of teeth and bone	Vitamin D, calcium, phosphorus	
Tooth pulp calcification		Vitamin D
Increased risk of candidiasis	Vitamins A, C, K, iron, zinc	
Decreased resistance to caries		Fluoride
Inadequate healing	Vitamin A, zinc	Vitamin A
Hypogeusia	Vitamins A, B_{12}, zinc	
Aphthous ulcers	Folic acid, vitamin B_{12}	

mouth rinses of chlorhexidine prostaglandin, glutamine, sucralfate, CM-CSF, camomile or allopurinol) prevented mucositis, but there is some evidence for the use of ice chips five minutes before and during an infusion of chemotherapy. The studies using ice are in adults with solid tumours receiving 5-flurouracil; any benefit may be through mucosal cooling decreasing blood flow locally and/or decreased cellular uptake of the drug at the time of peak circulating levels.

Treatment of chemotherapy induced mucositis As there is no definitive treatment of chemotherapy induced mucositis, the condition must be managed through meticulous oral hygiene, palliation of symptoms, and early treatment of infections. Mucositis when uncomplicated by secondary infection is self-limiting. Protocols often suggest a stepped approach, depending on the severity using a combination of the following:

(1) frequent rinses with 0.9% saline and/or sodium bicarbonate solution for oral lubrication and to stimulate saliva flow;

(2) regular lip care;

(3) benzydamine hydrochloride prior to meals;

(4) topical antimicrobial/antifungal rinses such as chlorhexidine aqueous;

(5) mucosal coating agents, for cytoprotectant and analgesic effects (antacids, kaolin solutions, and sucralfate);

(6) topical local anaesthetics and analgesics (see pain section).

The Cochrane review of interventions for treating oral mucositis in patients with cancer receiving chemotherapy and/or radiotherapy found little of benefit. Single trials reported allopurinol mouthwash and vitamin E as helpful for 5-fluouacil mucositis. Benzydamine hydrochloride, sucralfate, tetrachlorodecaoxide, chlorhexidine, and 'magic' (lignocaine solution, diphenhydramine hydrochloride, and aluminium hydroxide suspension) were not found to be effective.

Many medications have been incorporated into protocols or used in trials. Some benefit has been reported for aciclovir and pilocarpine in specific instances:

- *Aciclovir*: studies showed that patients who received additional aciclovir as prophylaxis to prevent herpes simplex virus reactivation, tolerated 50% more of the dose of etoposide, as severe mucositis was reported less often as the dose-limiting factor.

- *Pilocarpine*: in a small double-blind, placebo-controlled, randomized-controlled trial, mucositis occurred in fewer patients treated with pilocarpine than with placebo.

- *Chamomile* is said to have anti-inflammatory effects as well as promoting granulation and epithelialization but there is no evidence to support its use.

Cytoprotectants:

- *Sucralfate* has a cytoprotective effect probably mediated by prostaglandin release. A recent randomized-controlled trial with 102 patients receiving either sucralfate or placebo, found a reduction of severe mucositis from 47 to 29% in the treatment group. As sucralfate is cheap and well-tolerated, it needs further evaluation.

- *Prostaglandin E1* and *E2* have cytoprotective actions and early studies were promising but there is a possible increased risk of herpes infections.

Mucosal cell stimulants:

- *Glutamine* as a nutrient for rapidly dividing cells and energy source of intestinal epithelium has had varying results.

- *Low-energy laser therapy* has been tried, to promote the proliferation of mucosal cells, but is unproven.

Immunomodulatory agents:

- *Granulocyte macrophage colony stimulating factor* (GM-CSF) and *granulo-cyte colony stimulating factor* (G-CSF) may shorten the duration of neutropenia when given parenterally but no benefit has been shown when used as a mouthwash.

- *Thalidomide* has shown benefit in resistant cases of aphthous ulceration in patients with HIV. The mechanism of action is unclear but may reduce the production of TNF-α.

It has been suggested human immunoglobulin may confer passive immunity reducing the severity of mucositis.

Radiotherapy The proliferation of most buccal cells follows a clear circadian rhythm, with most cells being in the mitotic state at 9 p.m.. Therefore, the radiotherapy should ideally be administered in the morning hours to avoid the most radiosensitive part of the cell cycle.

Infective complications of mucosal injury

Infective agents most often involved in mouth conditions are *Candida* species and herpes simplex virus (HSV). Good oral hygiene as described above will reduce the risk of oral infections.

General measures aimed at preventing exposure to infective agents have a role. These measures need to be tailored to the patient and risks involved for them at the stage of the illness, e.g. ward and home cleanliness, mouth, skin, and food hygiene. Detailed referenced guidelines are available for preventing infections in bone marrow transplant recipients, see references.

Patients who are neutropenic are frequently given antibiotics, antifungal and antiviral agents prophylactically, as the risks from systemic infection are so great. There does not appear to be randomized-control trial evidence for the use of antibiotics at present. Recent systematic reviews of prophylactic antifungal agents and the number of fungal infection related deaths have produced conflicting results.

Bacterial infection The gastro-intestinal tract is the major source of bacteria in immunocompromized patients. Of cases of septicaemia in neutropenic patients, 25–50% derive from oral colonizing bacteria. Oropharyngeal mucositis is a statistically significant independent risk factor for septicaemia and several prospective studies highlight an increased risk of septicaemia with increasing severity of oral mucositis.

A generalized mucosal erythema may be due to bacteria, particularly staphylococci and coliforms. An oral swab or phosphate-buffered saline rinse may be required to identify the causative agent. A pseudomembranous inflammatory reaction may be caused by chemical irritants or bacteria (streptococci, staphylococci, gonococci, *Corynebacterium diphtheria*). Streptococci viridans and enterococci species are associated with systemic infections of oral origin in myelosuppressed patients.

The incidence of neutropenia-associated Gram-negative bacterial infections has decreased as a result of both the prophylactic use of antibiotics and the use of them empirically at fist signs of fever in neutropenic patients.

Gram-positive bacteria now represent the overwhelming majority of neutropenic systemic infections. Streptococcus viridans is now the second most common cause (isolated from blood cultures in about 35%) after coagulase-negative staphylococci. Several authors consider the oropharynx the most likely source of these streptococci, though others suggest the stomach or the respiratory tract. Most neutropenic patients with anaerobic bacteraemia have oral mucositis or periodontal disease.

Management Topical therapy includes chlorhexidine oral rinses, effervescent (peroxide) agents, or povidone iodine mouthwashes (as iodine is absorbed, therefore it is for short-term use only). Systemic treatment is necessary if the patient is immunocompromised. Microbiological identification and the establishment of sensitivities should guide the choice of antibiotic. However, in most neutropenic patients, cultures remain sterile and the treatment is empirical.

Fungal infection Oral candidiasis is a common condition and predisposing factors include:

(1) immunosuppression from disease or treatment; and

(2) the mucosal environment, i.e. xerostomia, antibiotics, malnutrition, high sugar levels, and dentures.

A significant proportion of patients undergoing BMT develop invasive fungal infection when neutropenia persists for more than 20 days. Antibiotics used during prolonged neutropenia alter the oral flora, encouraging fungal overgrowth that may be exacerbated by concurrent steroid therapy. In patients undergoing chemotherapy for leukaemia and in BMT-patients, *Candida* and *Aspergillus* sub-species are the most frequent causes of fungal infections. *Candida* sub-species. are commensal organisms of the oral mucosa in about 30–50% of the general population and of the lumen of the gastro-intestinal tract. Other fungi or moulds (*Triclosporon, Fusarium*, and *Aspergillus* species) may cause opportunistic infections of the mouth but the threat to the patient is usually from systemic infections.

The most common *Candida* infection is pseudomembranous candidiasis ('thrush') situated on buccal mucosa, palate, and tongue. The patient complains of a tender mouth, rough mucosa, and an altered or metallic taste; on examination, soft white or cream plaques are seen, which are easily wiped off to leave a raw, bleeding surface. Diagnosis is usually made on the clinical appearance, although microbiological culture from a swab or an oral rinse culture may be helpful. Commercial kits are available for near-patient testing; biopsy specimens may be required in chronic hyperplastic forms to confirm the diagnosis.

Oral candidiasis can also be seen in an erythematous form without the characteristic white plaques. The patient complains of a sore mouth with dryness, often after a course of antibiotics. This erythematous candidiasis can take on a chronic form, particularly in denture wearers and treatment should involve the dentures as the fungi survive on the acryllic denture plate. Fungal resistance is an emerging problem in the same way as antibiotic resistance.

Local infection of the oral cavity can cause pain, but can also result in oesophageal candidiasis or systemic dissemination. Systemic infection is difficult to diagnose and responds poorly to treatment, thus carrying a high mortality rate of 50–90%.

Mucosal injury facilitates fungal infection by facilitating adherence factors, allowing proliferation and translocation of microorganisms colonising these surfaces.

Management Preventative measures should take account of any predisposing factors. A Cochrane review found nystatin could not be recommended for prophylaxis and treatment of candida infections in immunosuppressed patients (7 or 12 trials reviewed were in patients with leukaemia), although some patients found the oral solution very soothing for palliation of symptoms. Another Cochrane review of interventions for preventing oral candidiasis found evidence for the use of antifungals that are absorbed (fluconazole) or partially absorbed (clotrimazole) in patients with cancer receiving chemotherapy.

Superficial candidiasis can usually be treated with fluconazole, or for a wider spectrum with itraconazole (against *Candida krusei* and *Candida glabrata*) or partially absorbed antifungals such as clotrimazole. Treatment should continue for at least 48 hours after symptoms have gone and many sources recommend treating for 10 to 14 days.

Viral infection Herpes simplex virus type 1 (HSV-1) is the most common cause for oral viral infection. Latent infection may be reactivated with chemo- or radiotherapy. The risk for reactivation correlates with the dose intensity of the antineoplastic treatment and occurs in up to 70–80% of HSV-seropositive BMT and acute leukaemia patients.

Infection with HSV can cause oral mucositis, which is indistinguishable from mucositis as a direct cause of chemotherapy, as the pathognomonic labial blisters are not necessarily present. Deep and extensive oral ulcers are often present and oesophagitis, tracheitis and pneumonitis can follow.

Other viruses causing mouth problems are cytomegalovirus (CMV), either new or reactivated and reactivated varicella zoster.

Management The incidence of HSV-related infections has been reduced with prophylactic aciclovir in seropositive patients. Prompt treatment with aciclovir (valaciclovir and famciclovir) is required to avoid dissemination. Other viruses causing mouth problems are cytomegalovirus (CMV), either new or reactivated, and reactivated varicella zoster. Infection with CMV can be treated with ganciclovir. Varicella-related disease requires aciclovir and famciclovir for systemic dissemination rather than oral disease. Acyclovir prophylaxis can also have secondary benefits as it reduces the risk of systemic infection from streptococcal bacteria colonizing the mucosa.

References

1 Eilers, J., Berger, A. M., and Peterson, M. C. (1988). Development, testing, and application of the Oral Assessment Guide. *Oncol Nurs Forum*, 1, 325–30.
2 Schubert, M. M., Williams, B. E., Lloid, M. E. *et al.* (1992). Clinical assessment scale for the rating of oral mucosal changes associated with bone marrow transplantation. *Cancer*, 69, 2469–77.

Further reading

Chiara, S., Nobile, M. T., Vincenti, M. *et al.* (2001). Sucralfate in the treatment of chemotherapy-induced stomatitis: a double-blind, placebo-controlled pilot study. *Anticancer Res*, 21(5), 3707–10.

Clarkson, J. E., Worthington, H. V., and Eden, O. B. (2000). Prevention of oral mucositis or oral candidiasis for patients with cancer receiving chemotherapy (excluding head and neck cancer). *Cochrane Database Syst Rev*, 2, CD000978.

Clarkson, J. E., Worthington, H. V., and Eden, O. B. (2002). Interventions for treating oral candidiasis for patients with cancer receiving treatment. *Cochrane Database Syst Rev*, 1, CD001972.

Sweeney, M. P. and Bagg, J. (2000). The mouth and palliative care. *Am J Hospice & Pall Care*, 17, 118–24.

Wilkes, J. D. (1998). Prevention and treatment of oral mucositis following cancer chemotherapy. *Seminars Oncol*, 25(5), 538–51.

Worthington, H. V., Clarkson, J. E., and Eden, O. B. (2992). Interventions for treating oral mucositis for patients with cancer receiving treatment. *Cochrane Database Syst Rev*, 1, CD001973.

J Natl Cancer Inst Monogr 2001; 29. The entire monograph is dedicated to the pathogenesis, latest research and new lines of management of treatment-induced mucositis in cancer patients.

Useful websites

Useful comprehensive website on mouth care: http://cancerweb.ncl.ac.uk/cancernet/302904.html.

The British Society for Disability and Oral Health has produced guidelines and standards on oral health in various groups of patients, including those critically and terminally ill. *The Essence of Care* published by the Department of Health is a practical toolkit for nursing care and includes a section on personal and oral hygiene. http://www.doh.gov.uk/essenceofcare/foreword.htm

A useful website giving detailed referenced guidelines for preventing infections in bone marrow transplant recipients: http://www.guideline.gov.

The dental faculty of the Royal College of Surgeons has produced guidelines for dental treatment of patients undergoing chemotherapy, radiotherapy and bone marrow transplants: http://www.rcseng.ac.uk/dental/fds/clinical_guidelines/

Chapter 8

The essentials of symptom control in haemato-oncology

Anna Spathis

Introduction

The goal of palliative care is achievement of the best possible quality of life for patients and their families.[1] Good symptom control is fundamental to palliative care, and provides enormous potential to improve quality of life.

In haemato-oncology, unlike in other malignancies, the disease is often potentially curable. Although palliative care has historically been provided for incurable disease, patients with haematological malignancy may still have considerable palliative care needs. Such patients are often symptomatic; they are treated aggressively, and a high proportion die in hospital. Hospital palliative care teams have an important role, but must appropriately adapt their management when caring for potentially curable patients. Control of distressing symptoms is still vital, even when the primary aim is cure of the disease.

Patients with haematological malignancy may experience symptoms both due to the disease and its treatment. This chapter will provide a practical overview of the assessment and management of such symptoms. There is little published evidence specific to symptom control in haemato-oncology; this chapter is based mostly on evidence extrapolated from studies in patients with other advanced cancers.

Principles

Principles of symptom control

Specific principles apply to the assessment and management of symptoms.

- **Aim to find the cause** of the symptoms. This aids appropriate management, particularly when the underlying cause is reversible.
- **Be proactive.** Ask direct questions and observe; do not wait for the patient to complain.

- **Treat promptly.** Neglected symptoms deteriorate, become harder to manage, and cause unnecessary distress.

- **Prescribe regularly.** Management of persistent symptoms with 'as needed' medication causes unnecessary suffering.

- **Reassess repeatedly** until symptom-free. Regular review is required to accurately titrate medication and to monitor for adverse effects.

- **Make one change at a time,** wherever possible. It is then easier to establish which changes have been useful.

Palliative care principles

These are also essential to achieve good symptom control.

- **Consider psychosocial and spiritual factors.** These can alter the perception of symptoms; anxiety and family tensions can, for example, worsen pain. Addressing a mistaken belief that the symptom reflects recurrent disease may help more than pharmacological intervention.

- **Good communication and 'patient-centred' care.** Listening to the patient's concerns, careful explanation, and involvement of patients in decision-making, can all aid the control of symptoms.

- **Multidisciplinary teamwork.** Colleagues can contribute to the control of complex symptoms. Examples include psychologists, anaesthetists, physiotherapists, and chaplains.

- **Attention to detail.** This is essential at every stage of assessment and management.

- **There is never 'nothing more that can be done'.** This phrase not only contributes to a perception of isolation and rejection, but is also generally untrue. Even with incurable disease it is invariably possible to ease suffering to some degree. If one strategy fails, try another one.

Common symptoms

The most common symptoms in haematological malignancy are pain, anorexia, constipation, nausea and insomnia (Table 8.1).[2] The following symptoms will be considered in some detail:

- pain
- nausea and vomiting
- constipation
- diarrhoea
- anorexia

Table 8.1 Prevalence of common symptoms in haemato-oncology

	Haemoto-oncology (%)	All cancer sites (%)
Pain	53	57
Anorexia	28	30
Constipation	20	23
Nausea	16	21
Insomnia	15	9
Dyspnoea	7	19

+ dyspnoea
+ excess secretions
+ anxiety
+ depression
+ insomnia.

Pain

Patients with haematological malignancy often have complex pain problems. They can suffer from bone and neuropathic pain, mouth pain from mucositis, and 'total pain'. These may not be particularly opioid-responsive and can be difficult to manage. Furthermore, simple analgesia such as paracetamol and NSAIDs may be contra-indicated after chemotherapy or in the presence of thrombocytopaenia. These difficulties will be addressed in detail in Chapter 9, whereas this chapter will provide an overview of the fundamentals of pain control.

Definitions

Pain is an unpleasant sensory and emotional experience associated with actual or potential tissue damage.[3]

Nociception is the perception of a painful stimulus by the nervous system; pain is the personal experience of this. It is a psychosomatic phenomenon affected by mood, morale, and the meaning the pain has for the patient. The term 'total pain', first used by Dame Cicely Saunders, encompasses the multiple dimensions of pain. Physical, psychological, social, and spiritual elements all contribute to patients' suffering.

Assessment

Most patients with haematological malignancy have more than one pain. The main aims of the assessment are to try to establish the **cause** and the **type** of each pain.

Determining the cause of the pain is central to effective treatment. Reversing the underlying cause is often more effective than analgesia alone. Establishing the type of the pain aids appropriate analgesic selection. Types of pain include visceral pain, soft tissue pain, bone pain, neuropathic pain, and muscle spasm. These vary in their responsiveness to morphine. Visceral pain, for example, is likely to respond to morphine. Neuropathic pain, bone pain and muscle spasm tend to respond less well.

History

A detailed history is crucial. The following elements are particularly important in a patient with cancer:

Character and temporal pattern The quality of the pain and its variation over time can help determine the type of pain. This may enable difficult, less morphine-responsive pains to be identified early. Bone pain and neuropathic pain are often worse on movement. Bone pain may be described as aching or throbbing, whereas neuropathic pain may be burning, stabbing or shooting in nature, and associated with abnormal sensation.

Exacerbating and relieving factors These can also help establish the type of pain. Rapidly progressive back pain exacerbated by sudden movements and partially relieved by sitting or standing, may be a sign of impending spinal cord compression, a problem that may occur in patients with myeloma or lymphoma.

Response to analgesia Many patients will have already tried analgesics. Detailed questioning is needed to find out which drugs have been tried, and with what beneficial and adverse effects.

Psychosocial and family history This may reveal factors exacerbating the pain, which may be contributing to 'total pain'. Severe pain may disrupt sleep and cause insomnia, anxiety and depression.

Patient's interpretation of the pain Misconceptions add to the patient's suffering. The patient's insight and understanding can also be ascertained.

Examination and investigations

These are vital to assess pain accurately. An area of tenderness over a bone in a patient with myeloma may, for example, suggest a lytic lesion. This could be confirmed on X-ray.

Management

Treatment of reversible causes

It may be possible to treat the underlying pathological process that is causing the pain. Examples include antibiotics for cellulitis, surgical fixation for a pathological fracture, and chemotherapy for disease suppression.

Analgesia

The principles of analgesic use are as follows:

◆ **Prescribe regularly.** In addition, 'as needed' medication should be prescribed for breakthrough pain.
◆ **Use the oral route.** This is appropriate for the majority of patients. If inadequate analgesia is achieved, consider using an alternative analgesic or a higher dose, rather than changing route. An equianalgesic parenteral dose is generally no more effective (unless there is a contraindication to the oral route, such as vomiting).
◆ **Use the three-step analgesic ladder** (Fig. 8.1). If a drug fails to relieve pain, move to the next step up the ladder, rather than to an alternative drug on the same step.
◆ **Monitor frequently.** Any benefit or adverse effects can then be detected.

Non-opioids The main non-opioids are paracetamol and NSAIDs. These drugs can be used at all three step of the analgesic ladder. They can contribute to pain control, even in combination with a strong opioid. Because of their anti-inflammatory effect, NSAIDs are particularly useful for bone and soft tissue pain. NSAIDs are inhibitors of both COX-1 and COX-2, the former resulting in many of the adverse effects, and the latter in most of the anti-inflammatory action. Selective COX-2 inhibitors have been developed to try to reduce NSAID adverse effects, in particular peptic ulceration. In practice, although there is a lower incidence of peptic ulcers, significant complications remain.

Use of these drugs in patients with haematological malignancy may, however, be limited by several factors:

◆ paracetamol and NSAIDs may mask pyrexia in neutropenic patients;
◆ in myeloma, renal function is often impaired, preventing safe use of NSAIDs;
◆ thrombocytopaenia, due to disease or chemotherapy, is also a contraindication to NSAIDs.

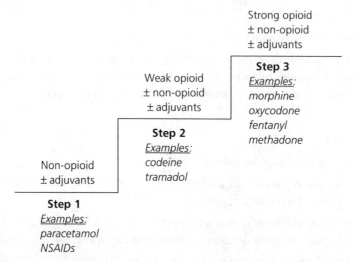

Strong opioid
± non-opioid
± adjuvants

Step 3
Examples:
morphine
oxycodone
fentanyl
methadone

Weak opioid
± non-opioid
± adjuvants

Step 2
Examples:
codeine
tramadol

Non-opioid
± adjuvants

Step 1
Examples:
paracetamol
NSAIDs

Opioids are agonists at endogenous opioid receptors, such as the mu receptor, producing 'morphine-like' activity.

Adjuvants are additional drugs that can be used as part of pain management, such as secondary analgesics (eg. gabapentin for neuropathic pain) and drugs to control analgesic adverse effects.

Weak opioid is an opioid for mild to moderate pain.

Strong opioid is an opioid for moderate to severe pain.

Fig. 8.1 World Health Organization three-step analgesic ladder.

Adjuvants These can be used at any of the three steps of the analgesia ladder.

♦ **Secondary analgesics.** These drugs may contribute to pain relief in certain situations. Tricyclic anti-depressants, anti-convulsants, and corticosteroids can help neuropathic pain. Muscle relaxants may be of benefit in pain from muscle spasm.

♦ **Control of analgesic adverse effects.** Laxatives and anti-emetics may be needed to counter the adverse effects of opioids.

Weak opioids Weak opioids have the same effect as a small dose of morphine. They are generally easier to obtain and supply than morphine, and are widely used. If a weak opioid is inadequate when given regularly, change to a strong opioid rather than to another weak one. Options include:

♦ **Codeine.** This is mainly a pro-drug of morphine. A proportion of the population (7% of Caucasians) are unable to make this conversion, codeine therefore lacking significant analgesic effect. It is about one-tenth as potent as morphine, and is very constipating.

♦ **Dihydrocodeine.** This is a semi-synthetic analogue of codeine that is virtually equipotent when taken orally.

- **Tramadol**. Potency is one-fifth that of morphine, and can therefore be considered as double-strength codeine. It causes significantly less constipation and respiratory depression than equianalgesic doses of morphine.

- **Compound preparations**. These include co-codamol, co-dydramol, and co-proxamol, which are combinations of paracetamol with codeine, dihydrocodeine, and dextropropoxyphene, respectively.

Strong opioids Morphine is the oral strong opioid of choice, mainly for reasons of familiarity, availability and cost.

- It is available in many forms, both normal release (e.g. in the UK, Oramorph and Sevredol, 4-hourly administration) and modified release (e.g. MST 12-hourly, and MXL 24-hourly administration).

- The **starting dose** is 2.5–5 mg normal-release morphine 4-hourly in an opioid naïve patient, and 5–10 mg normal-release morphine 4-hourly in a patient previously on a weak opioid. This should be prescribed regularly with the same dose as needed for breakthrough pain. The dose can be slowly titrated up according to the response. It is generally easier to start with normal-release morphine, and then convert to modified-release morphine once the dose has stabilized. To convert to MST, for example, the morphine requirement over 24 h (including 'as needed' doses) is added up and then divided by 2 to calculate the 12-hourly MST dose.

- The **route** used should be oral, unless the patient cannot take drugs by mouth. Parenteral morphine usually has no greater efficacy than an equianalgesic dose of oral morphine. If the parenteral route is needed, subcutaneous diamorphine is the strong opioid of choice in cancer pain. It is more soluble than morphine, and can therefore be dissolved in a smaller volume.

- **Adverse effects** include constipation, nausea, dry mouth, and drowsiness. All patients on strong opioids should be prescribed a regular laxative. Tolerance develops to the nausea, which tends to settle within days, but not to the constipation. Hallucinations, confusion and myoclonic jerks occur in opioid toxicity.

When used for pain, morphine does not result in clinically significant respiratory depression or addiction.

Alternative strong opioids These can be used if intolerable adverse effects to morphine develop before adequate analgesia is achieved (Table 8.2).

Adverse effects can differ to that of morphine. Fentanyl is significantly less constipating. Oxycodone is associated with a lower incidence of hallucinations.

Table 8.2 Comparison of alternative strong opioids with morphine

	Advantages	Disadvantages	Conversion calculation	Example of calculation
Diamorphine	Highly soluble in small volume. Suitable for parental route	Rarely used by oral route in UK, and not available outside the UK and Belgium.	Divide oral (po) morphine dose by three for subcutaneous (sc) diamorphine dose.	30 mg morphine po ≡ 10 mg diamorphine sc.
Oxycodone	May cause less nausea, pruritis and hallucinations.	New to the UK.	Divide oral morphine dose by two for oral oxycodone dose.	20 mg morphine po ≡ 10 mg oxycodone po.
Fentanyl	Significantly less constipating. Patch provides useful topical alternative to oral route. Less toxicity in renal failure.	Rapid titration is difficult. Less dose flexibility as only 25,50,75 and 100 μg/h patches available.	Divide patch size (in μg/h) by five for *4-hourly* sc diamorphine dose (in mg).	For a 25 μg/h fentanyl patch, the dose for breakthrough pain (equivalent to a 4-hourly dose) is 5 mg diamorphine sc or 15 mg morphine po. Therefore, 25 μg/h patch ≡ 90 mg morphine po in 24 h.

Before switching opioid, alternative measures can be tried:

◆ reduce the morphine dose

◆ use non-opioid and adjuvants to improve pain control

◆ treat the adverse effects, e.g. haloperidol can help nausea and hallucinations.

Dose calculations are summarized in Table 8.2. Until very familiar with the calculations, it is recommended that all calculations are checked against standard conversion charts. If in doubt about the dose the patient requires, prescribe below the calculated dose, and then titrate upwards.

Difficult pains Bone pain, neuropathic pain, and 'total pain' are examples of difficult pains, in that they are generally less responsive to morphine. Bone and neuropathic pain are often much worse on movement, causing 'incident pain'. Sufficient morphine to render a patient pain-free on movement may be excessive at rest, causing intolerable adverse effects. These pains will be described in greater detail in Chapter 9.

◆ **Bone pain** tends to respond well to NSAIDs. These should be used with caution in neutropenic or thrombocytopenic patients.

◆ **Neuropathic pain** may need adjuvant analgesia including an anticonvulsant (e.g. gabapentin), or an anti-depressant (e.g. amitriptyline). Local nerve blocks may help.

◆ **'Total pain'** may require specialized psychological or psychiatric input.

Difficult pains may all benefit from non-pharmacological measures.

Non-pharmacological methods

These include both physical and psychological methods. Psychological care should run as a thread through all patient care, but sometimes specific techniques and specialist psychological interventions are needed to help pain control. Multidisciplinary input may be required.

Physical interventions include:

◆ TENS-Transcutaneous Electrical Nerve Stimulation

◆ heat pads

◆ local anaesthetic or neurolytic nerve blocks.

Specific psychological interventions include:

◆ relaxation techniques

◆ cognitive behavioural therapy.

Nausea and vomiting

Nausea and vomiting are distressing symptoms, often inadequately managed. There are many potential causes in patients with haematological malignancy. Chemotherapy induced nausea and vomiting is relatively common in such patients, and the management of this will be considered in detail in Chapter 6. Here, the essentials of the management of nausea and vomiting of all causes will be described.[4]

Definitions

Nausea is the unpleasant feeling of needing to vomit. In can be associated with autonomic symptoms, including sweating, salivation, tachycardia, and diarrhoea. Retching occurs in the presence of nausea, and can lead to vomiting.

Vomiting is the forceful expulsion of gastric contents through the mouth. It is a primitive mechanism intended to protect the body from the ingestion of harmful substances.

Assessment

The main aim of the assessment is to establish the likely cause of the symptoms. This not only allows reversible causes to be appropriately managed, but aids the selection of the most appropriate anti-emetic.

History

It is very important to make a detailed evaluation of the nausea and vomiting. This should include:

- separate evaluation of the nausea and the vomiting
- severity, frequency, and diurnal variation of symptoms
- presence of nausea before and after vomiting
- triggering and relieving factors
- associated symptoms.

The clinical picture of the nausea and vomiting may give clues as to the underlying cause.[5]

Chemical causes For example, opioids, chemotherapy, uraemia:

- nausea is often particularly severe and persistent
- vomiting provides little or short-lived relief from the nausea.

Gastro-intestinal causes For example, gastric stasis, bowel obstruction:

- vomiting predominates
- little or intermittent nausea improved by vomiting

- vomitus may be of large volume, containing undigested food
- associated symptoms in bowel obstruction may include colicky pain, abdominal distension, and constipation.

Intracranial causes For example, brain metastases:
- may be associated with headache
- diurnal variation of symptoms may exist, with early morning predominance
- further evidence of possible underlying causes can be established from the rest of the history. A detailed drug history is particularly important.

Examination and investigations

Mouth, pharyngeal, and abdominal examination may contribute to assessment of the underlying cause. Investigations such as plasma concentrations of calcium, urea, creatinine, and radiological imaging may also be of use.

Management

Correct reversible causes

- **Drugs.** These are a common iatrogenic cause of nausea and vomiting. This occurs through several mechanisms that include gastric irritation (e.g. NSAIDs), gastric stasis (e.g. opioids, anticholinergics), and direct stimulation of the chemoreceptor trigger zone in the brainstem (e.g. opioids, digoxin, antibiotics).
- **Hypercalcaemia.** This is an often missed, but relatively easily correctable cause of nausea.
- **Raised intracranial pressure.** High-dose corticosteroids may be of benefit.
- **Severe pain.** Improving pain control may help not only the pain, but also nausea and vomiting.
- **Anxiety.** Nausea and vomiting can cause and be caused by anxiety. The resulting 'vicious cycle' can be broken if anxiety is reduced.
- **Tense ascites.** The functional bowel obstruction caused by ascitic pressure can be relieved by paracentesis or diuretics.
- **Coughing.** This can lead to retching and then vomiting. Treating the underlying cause of the cough, may also improve vomiting.

Non-drug measures

Avoiding exposure to foods that may trigger nausea, and control of malodour, such as from a fungating wound, may help nausea significantly. There is some evidence for the use of acupuncture. Simple measures to curb anxiety are important, such as a calm, reassuring environment and relaxation techniques.

Drug treatments

Knowledge of the cause of the symptom may aid selection of the most appropriate anti-emetic. Details of anti-emetic drugs, including indications, mechanism, and dose are shown in Table 8.3.

First-line anti-emetics The three most commonly used first-line drugs and their main indications, are as follows:

- metoclopramide
  - gastric stasis
  - functional bowel obstruction
- haloperidol
  - chemical causes such as drugs and renal failure
- cyclizine
  - mechanical bowel obstruction
  - raised intracranial pressure
  - movement related symptoms.

Principles of anti-emetic use

- Start with a first line drug, selecting according to the most likely cause of the nausea and vomiting.
- Re-evaluate regularly.
- If the first selected drug is ineffective, consider an alternative first-line anti-emetic, or a combination of first-line anti-emetics (such as haloperidol and cyclizine).
- Avoid prescribing a prokinetic anti-emetic with an anticholinergic drug concurrently, e.g. metoclopramide and cyclizine; the latter blocks the prokinetic action.
- Prescribe parenterally if vomiting is preventing enteric drug absorption. Nausea causes gastric stasis, and may therefore also hinder absorption of anti-emetics. Once good symptom control is achieved consider converting back to the oral regimen.
- Prescribe anti-emetics regularly and the same or an alternative anti-emetic as required.
- If nausea or vomiting persists, consider adding or substituting a second-line drug.

Table 8.3 Anti-emetic drugs

Drug	Indications	Mechanism of action	Dose	Comments
Metoclopramide	Functional bowel obstruction. Gastric stasis. Gastritis.	Prokinetic. D_2 antagonist + $5HT_4$ agonist. Prokinetic cholinergic nerves from myenteric plexus are inhibited by dopamine and stimulated by 5HT.	10 mg tds, po. 30 mg/24 h CSCI.	Effect blocked by antimuscarinic drugs, e.g. cyclizine. Combination of IV metoclopramide and IV ondansetron contra-indicated.
Haloperidol	Chemical causes of N + V including renal failure, drugs.	D_2 antagonist. Butyrophenone antipsychotic. Acts on chemoreceptor trigger zone, in area postrema, outside BBB.	1.5 mg on/bd, po. 5 mg/24 h CSCI.	Combines well with cyclizine. Useful in patients with anxiety, hallucinations, hiccups, etc. Sedating.
Cyclizine	Mechanical bowel obstruction. Raised intracranial pressure. Movement related N + V.	Antihistaminic and antimuscarinic. Acts on vomiting center, the central emetic pattern generator.	50 mg tds, po. 150 mg/24 h CSCI.	Can cause irritation at injection site. Can be sedating.
Hyoscine butylbromide	Mechanical bowel obstruction.	Antimuscarinic drug with both antispasmodic and antisecretory properties.	20 mg sc stat. 60–120 mg/24 h CSCI. Poorly absorbed po.	Not sedating as does not cross BBB. Useful in patients with bowel colic, excess respiratory secretions, etc.
Granisetron	Chemical causes of N + V. Situations of seratonin release e.g. bowel distension, abdominal RT and renal failure (from platelets).	$5HT_3$ antagonist.	1 mg od or bd, po or sc. Single sc dose lasts 24 h and therefore CSCI not needed.	Has advantages over ondansetron, in that only given once daily, and as effective po as sc. Constipating.
Levomepromazine	N + V of many causes.	Phenothiazine antipsychotic. Very broad spectrum: D_2, H_1, ACh, $5HT_2$ antagonist	6.25–6.25 mg od/bd, po/sc. 6.25–25 mg/24 h CSCI. Lasts 12–24 h (CSCI not necessarily needed).	'Nozinan' Usually substituted rather than added.
Dexamethasone	Multiple causes.	May reduce permeability of BBB to emetogenic substances. Anti-inflammatory effect.	4–8 mg od, po or sc.	Usually added to existing antiemetic regimen.
Octreotide	Mechanical bowel obstruction.	Synthetic somatostatin analogue. Reduces bowel secretions and increases fluid absorption.	250–600 µg/24 h CSCI.	Probably no more effective above 600 µg. Longer acting lanreotide now available (2 or 4 weekly injections).

N + V: nausea and vomiting. CSCI: continuous subcutaneous infusion. BBB: blood–brain barrier. RT: radiotherapy.

Second-line anti-emetics The choice of second line anti-emetic is again dependent on the likely cause of the symptoms (see Table 8.3). The following are usually *substituted* for a first line drug:

◆ levomepromazine—multiple causes

◆ granisetron—chemical causes

◆ hyoscine butylbromide—mechanical bowel obstruction.

Others can be *added* to existing regimens:

◆ dexamethasone—multiple causes

◆ octreotide—bowel obstruction.

Constipation

Patients with any advanced cancer, including haematological malignancies, may be prone to constipation. This may be caused by drugs, for example opioids, antimuscarinic drugs and 5HT3 antagonists. It may also be caused by the general debility of the disease; inactivity, poor nutrition, dehydration and weakness can all contribute to constipation.

Definitions

Constipation is the evacuation of stools less frequently than is normal for that particular individual. Some normal individuals open their bowels less than three times a week.

Faecal impaction is the accumulation of faeces in part of the bowel, usually the rectum, to form a firm mass, which is too large to be evacuated. This can result in overflow diarrhoea, abdominal pain, urinary retention and even bowel obstruction.

Assessment

The presence of constipation can be ascertained on history and examination of the abdomen and rectum. A rectal examination should generally not be performed in a neutropenic patient, because of the risk of sepsis. It is import-ant to remember that diarrhoea may be a sign of severe constipation. Abdominal masses that indent are more likely to be faeces rather than tumour. An abdominal X-ray may be necessary to diagnose high constipation when the rectum is empty.

Management

Non-pharmacological management

◆ Aim for a healthy, high fibre diet and increased fluid intake.

Table 8.4 Commonly used laxatives and rectal measures

	Stool softening predominates	Bowel stimulation predominates
Oral laxatives	Lactulose Liquid paraffin and magnesium hydroxide (Milpar) Movicol	Senna Co-danthramer Co-danthrusate Sodium picosulphate
Rectal measures	Arachis oil enema	Bisacodyl suppositories Glycerol suppositories

- Encourage activity.
- Avoid inhibition of the urge to defaecate. Rapid access to a toilet or commode is important.

Oral laxatives and rectal measures

These are either stool-softening, or bowel-stimulating (see Table 8.4). A combination of a softening and stimulating agent is often most effective. Bowel-stimulating drugs should be avoided if mechanical bowel obstruction is suspected. Some patients, particularly paraplegics and the very debilitated, may require rectal measures despite oral laxatives.

Diarrhoea

There are many potential causes of diarrhoea in patients with haematological malignancy. These include:

- infection, e.g. as a consequence of immunosuppressive chemotherapy
- drugs, e.g. chemotherapy, antibiotics, SSRIs, NSAIDs, excess laxatives
- overflow, e.g. due to constipation or partial bowel obstruction
- abdominal radiotherapy, causing a radiation enteritis.

Assessment

Careful assessment is essential to find the underlying cause and to determine any consequences of the diarrhoea, such as dehydration or electrolyte disturbances. This requires a detailed history, including all recent medication, and a clinical examination. Some investigations may be needed such as serum electrolytes, stool culture, and abdominal X-ray.

Management

Resuscitate

Rehydration and correction of electrolyte disturbances may be necessary.

Correct the underlying cause

Common examples include treatment of bacterial or fungal enteric infection, stopping diarrhoea-inducing drugs, and treatment of underlying constipation.

Anti-diarrhoeal medication

This may be required for symptom control while the underlying cause is being treated. Particular care must be made to exclude overflow diarrhoea. Options include:

- opioids, such as codeine, loperamide and morphine
- anti-secretory drugs, such as octreotide and hyoscine butylbromide, e.g. in intractable diarrhoea related to chemotherapy or graft versus host disease
- pancreatic enzyme replacement, such as creon capsules, in patients with pancreatic deficiency.

Anorexia

Loss of appetite has not only the physical consequences of weight loss and weakness, but also psychological and social sequelae. Patients and families may become anxious, fearing disease deterioration. Anorexia can contribute to patient isolation by leading to a loss of the social routine of meals, a routine that is already disrupted by life in hospital. There are many reversible causes of anorexia that must be considered. These include:

- nausea
- oral infection (e.g. candida)
- painful mouth (e.g. mucositis)
- oesophagitis
- dysphagia
- gastric stasis
- constipation
- drugs (e.g. cytotoxics)
- anxiety and depression.

Assessment

A detailed history and examination can determine both any reversible causes, and any consequences of the anorexia. Early satiety may be a symptom of gastric stasis.

Management

Manage reversible underlying causes

In haematological malignancy many causes are a consequence of intensive chemotherapy. Antifungal medication, pain relief for mucositis, and anti-emetics may help encourage oral intake. Metoclopramide is particularly useful if gastric stasis is suspected.

Pharmacological management

Corticosteroids (e.g. dexamethasone 4 mg od) and progestagens (e.g. medroxyprogesterone acetate 400 mg daily) can stimulate appetite. Progestagens take longer to work but have less potentially serious adverse effects. They are therefore more useful when the prognosis is longer.

Non-pharmacological management

Aim for attractive presentation of food and small portions. Availability of snacks encourages eating a little, often. A variety of food and experimentation to find preferred tastes is also important. Dietetic advice may be of help. Psychological support with reassurance and explanation may help to reduce anxiety. When the anorexia is due to the underlying disease rather than a reversible cause, naso-gastric or parenteral feeding does not improve weight or prognosis, and therefore has no role.

Dyspnoea

Dyspnoea is a particularly distressing symptom. As with other advanced cancers, there are many potential causes in patients with haematological malignancy:

♦ directly caused by the cancer, e.g. pleural effusions and massive ascites
♦ indirectly caused by the cancer, e.g. anaemia, pulmonary embolism, pneumonia, muscular weakness
♦ caused by treatment of the cancer, e.g. pulmonary fibrosis as a result of bleomycin and thoracic radiotherapy, and interstitial pneumonitis following a bone marrow transplant
♦ concurrent, non-malignant causes, e.g. asthma and cardiac failure.

Definition

Dyspnoea is an unpleasant perception of difficulty in breathing. It is a subjective sensation and can be strongly influenced by thoughts and feelings. Tachypnoea and hypoxia can be objectively measured, but do not correlate with dyspnoea.

Assessment

The main aim of the assessment is to establish the likely causes of the dyspnoea. In advanced disease, dyspnoea is frequently multi-factorial. A detailed history and full examination are mandatory; investigations such as CXR, oxygen saturation and PEFR may also be of benefit. The severity of dyspnoea can be determined by whether it occurs on exercise or at rest, and whether it disturbs sleep. An assessment of anxiety is also vital, as dyspnoea can both be a cause and a consequence of this. Ignoring this may result in a spiral of worsening dyspnoea and anxiety.

Management

Treat reversible causes

This is the priority. On a haematology ward, the majority of causes will be reversible. Blood transfusion for anaemia and antibiotics for infection are common examples.

Non-pharmacological treatment

These measures can be very effective and avoid the potential side-effects of drug treatment of dyspnoea. They can all be easily done on the ward.

- **Fan.** There is good evidence that facial cooling in the area served by the 2nd and 3rd branches of the trigeminal nerve can significantly reduce the sensation of breathlessness.[6] This is a simple, safe, cheap and can be portable.

- **Oxygen.** A number of studies show that oxygen can relieve breathlessness at rest in some patients, but that this does not correlate with the degree of hypoxia. It may be that the facial cooling provided by the stream of oxygen provides some of the benefit. The only way to predict who will benefit is by a trial of oxygen. However, in patients who are breathless on exertion, standardized exercise tests can be done, to assess oxygen saturations in air and at different concentrations of inhaled oxygen. Prevention of desaturation on exercise may be associated with increased exercise tolerance.

- **Breathing exercises.** By causing anxiety, dyspnoea can result in muscle tension, inefficient fast shallow breathing, and loss of control. Simple exercises can slow the rate of breathing by lengthening expiration time, encourage the use of the diaphragm and lower chest muscles, and help relax the muscles of the shoulders and upper chest. Physiotherapists commonly teach these exercises in the ward setting.

◆ **Relaxation therapy.** Simple exercises can help, such as progressive muscle relaxation and visualisation. Relaxing complementary therapies such as massage may also be of benefit.

◆ **Energy conservation.** Lifestyle adaptations, e.g. sitting in the shower, sleeping in a bed downstairs, and pacing activities, may all provide benefit.

Pharmacological treatment

Much drug treatment aims to manage the underlying cause of the dyspnoea, such as bronchodilators and steroids for bronchospasm. Two main classes of drugs directly reduce the perception of dyspnoea. These are useful when the underlying cause cannot be reversed.

◆ **Opioids.** There is good evidence that strong opioids reduce dyspnoea and may increase exercise tolerance;[7] nebulized opioids do not provide significant benefit

◆ **Benzodiazepines.** Despite conflicting evidence of efficacy in the literature, many patients report benefit with anxiolytic agents.

Opioids and benzodiazepines are respiratory depressants and therefore must be used with care, particularly in type 2 respiratory failure. Buspirone is a potentially useful non-benzodiazepine anxiolytic, which does not cause respiratory depression. However, it takes 2 to 3 weeks to produce a clinical effect.

Excess secretions

Patients who are extremely weak, including the moribund, may be unable to expectorate effectively. Respiratory secretions and saliva then oscillate in the upper airways during breathing, producing a characteristic noise. This is sometimes referred to as 'death rattle'.

Assessment

It is important to assess the likely cause of the excess secretions. If, for example, they are a consequence of pneumonia, they are less likely to respond to an anti-secretory drug. Antibiotics may provide some symptom control in this situation. Excessive use of nebulizers, particularly nebulized saline, may contribute to the secretions, and should ideally be stopped.

Management

Suctioning should generally be avoided as patients usually dislike it.

Explanation

The rattle produced by the secretions can be very distressing to relatives, and may be perceived by them as causing distress to the patient. Reassurance and explanation of the cause of the secretions often reduces their distress, and may avoid the need for drug treatment.

Anti-secretory drugs

Subcutaneous options include hyoscine butylbromide 20 mg stat or 20–40 mg/24 h by continuous infusion and glycopyrrolate 200 μg stat or 600 μg/24 h by continuous infusion. These drugs do not act centrally and are not sedating. Hyoscine hydrobromide 400 μg stat or 1.2 mg/24 h by continuous infusion is usually effective but sedating. Transdermal hyoscine hydrobromide is another option.

Anxiety

Anxiety is a common consequence of any illness. Patients with haematological malignancy are often young. They may be teenagers still living with their parents, or they may have young families of their own. Furthermore the disease often has a very unpredictable course, and may involve particularly intensive therapy with associated side-effects. All these situations can exacerbate anxiety.

Definition

Anxiety is an unpleasant state of experiencing apprehension or uneasiness. It may result in insomnia, irritability, sweating, nausea, and, if very severe, panic attacks. Causes include:

◆ uncontrolled symptoms such as pain, nausea and dyspnoea
◆ drugs, such as corticosteroids, SSRIs and neuroleptics, and also drug withdrawal such as from benzodiazepines
◆ fear of future situations, including potential symptoms and death
◆ a reflection of family anxiety.

Assessment

The symptom of anxiety is often ignored, as it is considered a normal reaction to a serious situation. However, it is important that anxiety is assessed in detail, as appropriate management provides enormous scope to improve patients' quality of life.

- Is it acute or long-standing?
- Are there specific fears?
- In what situations does it occur?
- Are there physical consequences including insomnia or panic attacks?
- Does the patient have an accurate understanding of their situation?

Management

Address the underlying cause

This may include improving symptom control and correcting misconceptions.

Psychological therapies

Options include relaxation therapies, creative therapies (such as art and music therapy), and counselling. Involvement of a psychologist may sometimes be necessary, for example, for cognitive-behavioural and psychodynamic therapies. A psychological approach to managing anxiety is often the most effective.

Pharmacological therapies

Medication side-effects and concerns about addiction and tolerance can limit the use of drugs. Options include:

- **Benzodiazepines.** Diazepam has a long half-life of over 24 h. A once daily dose is therefore adequate, and it may cause daytime drowsiness. Lorazepam and midazolam are other options with shorter half-lives.
- **Anti-depressents.** Although SSRIs can cause anxiety in some patients, paroxetine can be very useful in generalized anxiety. There is often co-existent depression. Amitriptyline has the advantage of aiding sleep at night.
- **Anti-psychotics.** Haloperidol can be particularly useful if there is associated paranoia.

Depression

A significant proportion of patients with advanced malignancy may become depressed; some figures suggest up to 40%. It is often under-recognized in this situation. Medical staff may ignore low mood considering it to be an 'understandable reaction', and symptoms such as weight loss, anorexia, and sleep disturbance can be attributed to the disease rather than depression. However, it is extremely important to diagnose, as management can be very effective.

Definition

It can be difficult to distinguish between depression and appropriate sadness. Features that particularly suggest depression include:

*   **anhedonia:** lack of interest or pleasure in anything, including things that would normally be enjoyed such as visits of grandchildren
*   **loss of all emotion:** patients may have a flat affect and be unable to express sad emotions as well as happy ones
*   **low self-esteem:** guilty ruminations, self-doubt and loss of confidence may occur
*   **diurnal variation:** symptoms can be worse in the morning than later in the day
*   **hopelessness:** this may be associated with persistent thoughts of death or suicide.

Assessment

The important point is that an assessment for depression must be made in all patients. Sometimes a simple direct question such as, 'Do you think you are depressed?' may be most fruitful. A more detailed history can help distinguish between depression and sadness.

Management

Explanation

Some patients feel that depression is a sign of weakness. An explanation in medical terms may make it easier for the patient to accept treatment.[8] It could be explained, for example, that 'the continued stress of being ill has depleted certain chemicals in the brain, which can be replenished by anti-depressants.'

Drugs

These can be extremely effective and, unlike in anxiety, there can be a low threshold for commencing drug treatment. The choice of anti-depressant may depend on the side-effect profile. A tricyclic anti-depressant, for example, may be started in patients with sleeping difficulties, but an SSRI would be more appropriate in a patient with a risk of urinary retention. Venlafaxine is effective in very severe depression. Anti-depressants may take weeks to reach full clinical effect. When the prognosis is short, there may be role for psycho-stimulant drugs such as methylphenidate (start on 2.5–5 mg od and titrate up to 5–10 mg bd).

Others

Psychological support and social integration are of benefit. In some patients, psychiatric referral may be necessary.

Insomnia

Insomnia is an enormously under-recognized symptom in advanced cancer. As with depression, it may be considered to be a normal reaction to the situation. Patients also under-report, and there is a lack of awareness amongst health professionals. The consequences are severe. Irritability, loss of concentration, fatigue, and muscle aches commonly occur. There is some evidence for immune down-regulation and increased mortality, although this has not been shown in patients with cancer. There is a wide range of potential causes:

♦ The disease can have a direct effect on brainstem pathways involved in sleep. This has been reported, for example, in cerebral lymphoma.[9]

♦ Uncontrolled symptoms may prevent sleep.

♦ The psychological response to the diagnosis may interfere with sleep. Anxiety and depression may occur.

♦ Hospitalization, with noisy wards and unfamiliar routines, can inhibit sleep.

♦ Drug therapy can affect sleep in many ways: corticosteroids cause insomnia, as does withdrawal from medication such as opioids and benzodiazepines.

Assessment

A detailed sleep history is needed to assess the possible causes. Details of sleep hygiene must also be determined (see below).

Management

Treat the underlying cause

For example, avoidance of corticosteroid doses after 2 p.m. can be of benefit.

Optimize sleep hygiene

This provides enormous scope to safely and easily improve insomnia.

Improve the sleep environment For example:

♦ provide a quiet and dark bedroom, neither too hot nor too cold;

♦ avoid using the bedroom for work, television, and so on.

Clearly the hospital ward is often a poor sleep environment. Patients in hot wards may spend the whole day in bed, and are then frequently woken at night for routine observations. Although difficult, it can be possible to improve the situation, e.g. minimizing nocturnal nursing observations.

Improve sleep–wake patterns For example:

- increase exercise, but not within three hours of sleep time
- avoid daytime naps
- regular, relaxing pre-sleep routine
- light snack or milky drink
- optimize bladder or bowel function.

Again this may not be easy in hospital. Ill patients may be unable to exercise, but where possible daily mobilization should be encouraged.

Change drug intake For example:

- avoid caffeine, alcohol and corticosteroids
- optimize diuretic timing.

Pharmacological management

Hypnotics should be chosen according to their duration of action. A drug with a short-half-life can be used for difficulty in sleep initiation, and one with a longer half-life for early morning awakening. Use is limited by tolerance and, particularly in the elderly, any 'hang-over' can result in, for example, falls.

Non-pharmacological management

Behavioural therapy can be very effective and is simple to explain. Examples include:

- **Stimulus control therapy.** This aims to condition the patient to associate being in bed with successful sleep. The patient should only go to bed when sleepy, and should get up if awake for 15–30 min. It is best to leave the bedroom and carry out a non-stimulating activity, only returning when feeling sleepy again.
- **Sleep restriction.** Again, this aims to reverse the negative conditioning that perpetuates insomnia, as sleep deprivation should lead to deeper more continuous sleep.[10]

Psychotherapy including mental relaxation and cognitive therapy may occasionally be needed.

Conclusions

The key to successful symptom control is to find the underlying cause of the symptom. This allows the management of reversible causes, and helps decide the most appropriate management. Early referral to a hospital palliative care team may contribute to successful control of symptoms, and also provide psychosocial support. Irrespective of whether the disease is curable, good symptom control can provide enormous scope for improving the quality of life of both patients and their families.

References

1 WHO Expert Committee (1990). Cancer pain relief and palliative care. *Technical Report Series*, No. 804.

2 Vainio, A. and Auvinen A (1996). Prevalence of symptoms among patients with advanced cancer: an international collaborative study. Symptom Prevalence Group. *Journal of Pain and Symptom Management*, 12(1), 3–10.

3 Merskey, H. and Bogduk, N. (1994). Classification of chronic pain. In *IASP task force on taxonomy*, pp. 209–14. IASP Press, Seattle.

4 Twycross, R. and Back, I. (1998). Nausea and vomiting in advanced cancer. *European Journal of Palliative Care*, 5(2), 39–45.

5 Bentley, A. and Boyd, K. (2001). Use of clinical pictures in the management of nausea and vomiting: a prospective audit. *Palliative Medicine*, 15, 247–153.

6 Schwarzstein, R. M., Lahive, K., Pope, A. *et al.* (1987). Cold facial stimulation reduces breathlessness induced in normal subjects. *Am Rev Respir Dis*, 136(1), 58–61.

7 Jennings, A. L., Davies, A. N., Higgins, J. P. T. *et al.* (2002). Opioids for the palliation of breathlessness in terminal illness (Cochrane review). *The Cochrane Library*, Issue 3.

8 Twycross, R. (1997). *Symptom management in advanced cancer*, p. 103. Radcliffe Medical Press, Oxon.

9 Spathis, A., Morrish, E., Booth, S. *et al.* (2002). Selective circadian rhythm disturbance in cerebral lymphoma. *Sleep Medicine* (In press).

10 Shneerson, J. (2000). Insomnia. In *Handbook of sleep medicine*, p. 86. Blackwell Science, Oxon.

Chapter 9

When the opioid fails: managing the patient with severe neuropathic pain

Annette Vielhaber and Russell K. Portenoy

Introduction

Pain is experienced by approximately 75% of cancer patients with advanced stage disease. Neuropathic mechanisms are involved in approximately 40% of cancer pain syndromes and can be disease-related (e.g. tumour invasion of nerve plexus) or treatment-related (e.g. chemotherapy-induced painful polyneuropathy). In populations with metastatic solid tumours, most neuro-pathic pain is related to the disease itself. Although populations with haemato-logical malignancies may have less pain overall,[1] neuropathic pain is relatively common, presumably due to the close proximity of lymph nodes and nerve plexus. Treatment-related neuropathic pain also is likely to be prevalent in this population given the observation that most patients with haematological malignancies die while receiving active treatment.[1,2]

Although neuropathic pain may respond well to opioids,[3] it is, overall, less responsive to opioids than pains due to other pathophysiologies.[6-8] Neuropathic pain that is poorly responsive to opioid therapy is a challenging clinical problem in patients with haematological malignancies.

Strategies to address the problem in this population may be developed, based on a growing scientific understanding of neuropathic pain in general and studies of treatments for neuropathic pain associated with other diseases. Some problems specific to patients with haematological malignancies, such as thrombocytopenia or neutropenia secondary to bone marrow infiltra-tion, have to be taken into account. Given their inhibitory effect on platelet aggregation, the use of non-steroidal anti-inflammatory drugs is often problematic in this population. Due to the risk of bleeding and infection, the placement of intra-spinal catheters is only indicated after a thorough risk–benefit analysis.

What is neuropathic pain?

Pain is labelled neuropathic if there is evidence that it is sustained by abnormal somatosensory processing in the peripheral or the central nervous system (CNS). Neuropathic cancer pain usually results from injury to peripheral nerves, which may be caused by tumour invasion, cancer treatment, or other factors (e.g. post-herpetic neuralgia). Any of numerous discrete mechanisms may be involved. In the periphery, for example, regenerating nerve sprouts at sites of axonal damage may discharge spontaneously or have markedly lower activation thresholds than uninjured nerve. In the CNS, the stimulus–response function of second-order neurons may shift to the left, such that a noxious stimulus causes more pain than normal (hyperalgesia) or non-noxious stimuli are perceived as painful (allodynia). This state of increased central neuronal activity is known as central sensitization.

Neuropathic pain is diagnosed on the basis of the patient's verbal description of the pain, typically frequently supported by evidence of nerve injury. Patients may use any of a variety of verbal descriptors but some, such as 'burning', 'shock-like,' or 'electrical', are particularly suggestive of neuropathic pain. Areas of abnormal sensations are often found on physical examination. These may include hypesthesia (a numbness or lessening of feeling), paresthesias (abnormal non-painful sensations such as tingling, cold, or itching), hyperalgesia (increased perception of painful stimuli), hyperpathia (exaggerated pain response), and allodynia (pain induced by non-painful stimuli, such as light touch, cool air).[10]

Examples of neuropathic pain syndromes in haematologic malignancies
Disease-related neuropathic pain syndromes

Involvement of vertebral bodies with extra-dural compression of the spinal cord or its nerve roots is an important complication of multiple myeloma. Similarly, proximal extension of para-spinal or retroperitoneal lymph nodes may lead to spinal cord compression or radiculopathy in lymphoma patients. Approximately 4% of lymphoma patients and 11% of myeloma patients develop spinal cord or cauda equina compression during the course of their respective illness. Progressive back pain or radicular pain, which may be aggravated by coughing, sneezing, or straining, may be a warning of impending cord or cauda injury and should be investigated by means of MRI.

Cervical, axillary, para-aortic, or retroperitoneal lymph nodes may infiltrate plexus resulting in cervical, brachial, or lumbosacral plexopathy. Pain is the most common symptom, followed by muscle weakness and sensory abnormalities.

Peripheral neuropathy is a classical complication of the paraproteinemias. In patients with Waldenström's macroglobulinemia, for example, 5–10% of patients develop neuropathy. The neuropathy usually manifests as a sensory syndrome with distal numbness, paresthesias, and reduced proprioception, and progresses gradually. Tremor, generalized areflexia, and gait ataxia are also common findings. Limb weakness develops in the majority of cases but rarely overshadows the sensory findings. Similarly, 3–5% of patients with multiple myeloma develop a progressive sensorimotor polyneuropathy; 50% are associated with amyloid.

Treatment-related neuropathic pain syndromes

In patients who have been treated with radiotherapy, the appearance of plexopathy may be due to the radiation and not to the underlying disease itself. Symptoms usually occur after a latent period of 6 months and the interval may be much longer, sometimes many years. Slowly progressing symptoms, electomyographic recording of myokymic discharges, and absence of a space-occupying mass in MRI-imaging studies, suggest radiation-induced plexopathy. Pain is usually milder than in disease-related plexopathy.

Chemotherapy-induced peripheral neuropathy usually improves after treatment stops, but can become a persistent problem for some patients. Pre-existing nerve damage, such as diabetic or alcoholic neuropathy, or disease-related peripheral neuropathy may add to the risk of chemotherapy-induced neuropathy.

Vincristine is crucial in the treatment part of haematological malignancies and is part of commonly used regimens such as VAD (vincristine, doxorubicin, dexamethasone) and CHOP (cyclophosphamide, doxorubicin, vincristine, prednisolone). Vincristine acts by binding on intra-cellular tubulin. In the peripheral nervous system the drug rapidly induces alterations in the microtubules, which leads to oedema in the fast and slow conducting axons. Most of the patients treated with vincristine develop a dose-dependent (>4 mg cumulative doses) primarily sensory neuropathy.[4] Early signs are paresthesias affecting the hands before the feet, dysesthetic pain, and loss of deep tendon reflexes. Muscle cramps and muscle weakness appear in more advanced stages. More than one-third of the patients develop signs of autonomic nervous system dysfunction, such as orthostatic hypotension and constipation. Most of these symptoms are reversible after months or years.[4]

Cisplatin is constituent of several treatment protocols for refractory or relapsed lymphomas, such as ESHAP (etoposide, methylprednisolone, high-dose cytarabine, and cisplatin) and DHAP (dexamethasone, cytarabine, and cisplatin). Cisplatin has a high affinity for the peripheral nervous system and can be detected in dorsal root ganglion cells and the sensory nerves themselves. It leads to loss of axons, with secondary atrophy of the dorsal root.

First signs of the predominately sensory neuropathy appear about one month after initiation of therapy. Cumulative doses above 400 mg/m^2 almost always lead to neuronal damage.[4]

Clinically, cisplatin-induced neuropathy is characterized by diminished vibration perception, loss of tendon reflexes and uncomfortable paraesthesias starting in the lower extremities. In advanced stages the patient may develop ataxic gait due to impaired proprioception. Motor nerves are normally spared. A specific feature of cisplatin-induced peripheral neuropathy is that symptoms may start even after cessation of therapy. Usually, symptoms decline over several months.[4]

Other neuropathic pain syndromes

Patients with cancer, especially haematological malignancies, have an increased risk of herpes zoster. Between 3 and 10% of lymphoma patients develop herpes zoster. The infection is more likely to occur in patients with advanced disease and those with iatrogenic immunosuppression from systemic chemotherapy, splenectomy or irradiation. According to a recent classification, acute herpetic neuralgia is pain during the first 30 days after the outbreak of the rash. Subacute herpetic neuralgia is the pain that resolves within 3 months following the initial illness. Post-herpetic neuralgia (PHN) is pain that persists 4 months or more. Reports of prevalence rates for PHN range from 9 to 34%. The proportion of patients who develop PHN is higher in those over 70 years old. Patients with PHN often describe a constant burning or ache, an intermittent lancinating component, and a dysesthetic or pruritic sensation. Allodynia, hyperesthesia, and hyperpathia may be present.

Treatment strategies for neuropathic pain poorly responsive to opioids

Pain is considered poorly responsive to opioids if it cannot be controlled with dose escalation because of moderate to severe opioid-related side-effects. Patients whose neuropathic pain has been opioid-responsive, but who experience either an increase in pain intensity or a change in pain quality, should first be comprehensively reassessed to determine whether specific contributing factors can be identified. Relapse or disease progression, for example, may be amenable to primary therapeutic strategies, such as chemotherapy to address disease progression associated with loss of analgesic effectiveness. Other conditions, such as cord compression, systemic, or local infection, and psychological distress (e.g. depression), also may be treatable.

The initial strategy to address the pain itself typically involves adjustment of the opioid regimen. Alternative strategies are needed if poor responsiveness is confirmed by the development of treatment-limiting side-effects as the opioid dose is increased. Four broad strategies can be considered:

(1) pharmacological approaches that may reduce the opioid requirement;

(2) a switch to a different opioid drug;

(3) more aggressive side-effect management; and

(4) non-pharmacological approaches to reduce the opioid requirement.[5]

The most dramatic recent advances in the area of neuropathic pain have occurred in the availability of pharmacological therapies that may reduce the opioid requirement. These include an expanding number of systemic drugs—the so-called adjuvant analgesics—and a greater role for neuraxial (intraspinal) drug infusion.

Primary therapy directed at the aetiology of the pain should be considered whenever assessment of the patient with poorly opioid responsive neuropathic pain suggests that such an approach is possible. Patients who suffer from pain during the course of a refractory or relapsed lymphoma or myeloma may benefit dramatically from palliative chemo- or radiotherapy.

Adjuvant analgesics

Adjuvant analgesics may be defined as drugs that are commercially available for indications other than pain but may be analgesic in selected circumstances. The pharmacological options available for neuropathic pain have advanced rapidly in recent years and clinical experience suggests that most patients with neuropathic cancer pain that is poorly responsive to an opioid can be managed through the addition of an adjuvant analgesic. In the cancer population, adjuvant analgesics may be important in the management of diverse syndromes and their use in neuropathic pain is now commonplace.

Very few of the adjuvant analgesics have been studied in the palliative care setting and the information used to develop dosing guidelines is usually extrapolated from other patient populations. Low initial doses and gradual dose escalation may avoid early side-effects and identify dose-dependent analgesic effects that can be explored to improve the balance between pain relief and adverse effects. The use of low initial doses and dose titration may delay the onset of analgesia, however, and patients must be informed about this possibility to improve compliance.

Corticosteroids

Given their anti-tumour and anti-inflammatory properties, corticosteroids may be particularly helpful in the treatment of neuropathic pain in patients with lymphoma-related plexopathy. Doses usually start with 5–10 mg prednisolone or 1–2 mg dexamethasone once or twice daily, and are then titrated as needed to achieve the best possible effect on the lowest effective dose. In selected patients with severe progressive pain related to spinal cord compression or nerve injury, a higher dose regimen may begin with intravenous dexamethasone at 20–100 mg, followed by 60–90 mg daily in three divided doses. This dose is tapered gradually while an alternative analgesic approach, such as radiation or neural blockade, is implemented.

Anti-convulsants

Originally, anti-convulsants were thought to be most effective in syndromes characterized by lancinating or paroxysmal neuropathic pain such as trigeminal neuralgia. Recent data, however, support their usefulness in a broad variety of neuropathic pain syndromes.

Evidence for analgesic efficacy is best for gabapentin, and this drug is now widely used for neuropathic pain of all types.

In two large controlled studies of patients with peripheral diabetic neuropathy and PHN, gabapentin was shown to be efficacious for the treatment of pain and pain-related interference with sleep, mood, and quality of life.[6,7]

In an uncontrolled study of 22 cancer patients whose neuropathic pain was not completely controlled with opioids, the addition of gabapentin resulted in a decrease of pain in 20 patients.[8] Gabapentin significantly reduced the pain in 48% of patients with chemotherapy induced peripheral neuropathy.

Gabapentin's mechanism of action is unknown. It is a chemical analogue of the ubiquitous inhibitory neurotransmitter GABA, but does not act as a GABA-receptor agonist. It binds to a receptor site in the CNS, a gabapentin-binding protein, and interacts with calcium channels, and increases GABA synthesis and release.

Gabapentin has an acceptable adverse effect profile, is not metabolized in the liver, and has no known drug–drug interactions. The most commonly seen side-effects include somnolence, dizziness, ataxia, and peripheral oedema. Treatment usually starts with 100–300 mg/day, and dose titration continues until benefit occurs, side-effects supervene, or the total daily dose is at least 2700–3600 mg/day (Table 9.1). Some patients do not reach a maximal response until the dose is increased to 6000 mg/day or even higher. A slow titration of the dose is recommended in patients who are elderly, have renal impairment, or are receiving other CNS depressant drugs. Dose adjustment is

Table 9.1 Dose escalation for gabapentin

Fast		Slow	
Day 1	300 mg at bedtime	Day 1	100 mg at bedtime
Day 2	300 mg bid	Day 4	100 mg tid
Day 3	300 mg tid	Day 7	300 mg tid
Day 4	400 mg tid	Day 14	600 mg tid
Then increase by 300 mg/day until benefit occurs, side effects supervene, or the total daily is at least 2700–3600 mg per day		Day 21	900 mg tid
		Day 28	1200 mg tid

Table 9.2 Anti-convulsants used as adjuvant analgesics

Drug	Usually effective daily dose	Doses per day	Evidence
Gabapentin	300–3600 mg/day (or higher)	1–4	CT
Carbamazepine	100–1600 mg/day	2–4	CT
Valproate	500–3000 mg/day	2	OLT
Phenytoin	100–300 mg/day	1–3	CT
Clonazepam	1–10 mg/day	1–3	OLT
Lamotrigine	150–500 mg/day	2	CT
Topiramate	25–400 mg/day	2	CT
Pregabalin	300–600 mg/day	1–2	CT
Oxcarbazepine	300–2400 mg/day	2	OLT

CT = controlled trials; OLT = open label trials; CR = case reports.

recommended in patients with renal impairment or those undergoing haemodialysis. The daily dose is usually administered in two to three equal parts, but if daytime sedation remains a problem, a single night-time dose can be used for analgesia and sleep-related benefits. Patients should not take antacids containing aluminium or magnesium within two hours of the gabapentin dose. If required, the capsules can be opened and the contents mixed with water, fruit juice, etc.

Other anti-convulsants also have established analgesic effects. Carbamazepine, phenytoin, valproate, and clonazepam have been used for many years. Despite its high effectiveness, the utility of carbamazepine in the cancer population is limited by its potential to produce bone marrow suppression in up to 7% of cases, and to alter liver metabolism of other drugs. A variety of observations, including several controlled trials, also support the potential efficacy of the newer anti-convulsants, including lamotrigine, topiramate, tiagabine, and oxcarbazepine (Table 9.2).

Sequential trials of different agents may be needed to identify the most useful agent. Clonazepam may be particularly useful if pain is associated with anxiety.

Anti-depressants

Anti-depressants have been found to be effective in a variety of neuropathic pain syndromes. Although widely accepted as adjuvant drugs, there have been no randomized trials of anti-depressants for cancer-related neuropathic pain (Table 9.3).

Tricyclic anti-depressants have been found to be effective in the treatment of PHN and peripheral diabetic neuropathy. A recent controlled study of 25 patients with peripheral diabetic neuropathy compared amitriptyline with gabapentin, finding no difference in pain relief or adverse effects. However, gabapentin is typically better tolerated.

Nortriptyline and desipramine may be effective and are better tolerated than amitriptyline. Adverse effects are even less likely with the selective serotonin re-uptake inhibitors (SSRI), but evidence of analgesic efficacy for these drugs is very limited. Several controlled studies, however, do suggest efficacy for drugs such as paroxetine.

Table 9.3 Anti-depressants used as adjuvant analgesics

Drug	Usually effective daily dose	Doses per day	Evidence
Tricyclic anti-depressants			
Tertiary amines			
Amitriptyline	10–300 mg	1	CT
Imipramine	10–300 mg	1	CT
Secondary amines			
Nortriptyline	10–150 mg	1	CT
Desipramine	10–300 mg	1	CT
Second- and third-generation agents			
Trazodone	50–400 mg	1–3	CR
Maprotiline	25–225 mg	1–2	CT
Selective serotonin re-uptake inhibitors			
Citalopram	20–80 mg	1	CT
Fluoxetine	20–80 mg	1	CT
Paroxetine	20–80 mg	1	CT
Sertraline	50–250 mg	1	OLT

CT = controlled trials; OLT = open-label trials; CR = case report.

Anti-depressants potentiate serotonin and/or noradrenaline in the CNS. These neurotransmitters are thought to be involved in pain-inhibiting systems descending from the brainstem to the dorsal horn of the spinal cord.

The use of tricyclics is limited by the high likelihood of side-effects. In a study of 15 patients with post-mastectomy syndrome treated with amitrypti-line, five of the eight women who had a good response did not want to continue due to adverse events (the order of importance being tiredness, dry mouth, and constipation).[10] Urinary retention, confusion, and orthostatic hypoten-sion are less common. Patients who have significant heart disease, including conduction disorders, arrhythmia, or heart failure, should not be treated with a tricyclic. The secondary amine tricyclic drugs are less anticholinergic and, therefore, better tolerated than the tertiary amines. They also are less likely to cause orthostatic hypotension, somnolence, and confusion. The SSRI are bet-ter tolerated than the tricyclic compounds. Common side-effects include insomnia, tremor, gastro-intestinal symptoms, and sexual dysfunction.

Amitriptyline is the most studied agent and, on this basis, it may be pre-ferred in patients with cancer-related neuropathic pain. However, the likeli-hood of severe adverse effects is so high that many patients are considered for a trial with a secondary amine tricyclic, such as nortriptyline or desipramine. A trial with paroxetine or another of the newer anti-depressants is appropriate for those who cannot tolerate a secondary amine tricyclic drug or have contra-indications to a tricyclic trial. If there is no benefit after dose escalation over several weeks, the anti-depressant should be discontinued. After a few weeks of treatment, it is prudent to taper the dose before stopping the treatment to reduce the likelihood of withdrawal symptoms such as insomnia.

Local anaesthetics

Intravenous lidocaine has been found to effectively alleviate neuropathic pain associated with painful diabetic neuropathy and PHN. Subcutaneous lidocaine has been shown to be effective in the treatment of cancer-related neuropathic pain. The oral local anesthetic mexiletine has been used in the treatment of a variety of neuropathic pain syndromes with mixed results. In a pilot study evaluating oral anesthetics for the treatment of cancer-related neuropathic pain inadequately controlled with opioids, 90% of the patients did not benefit from mexiletine and many of the responders had intolerable nausea/gastro-intestinal distress.[11] In a small prospective study, pain relief following an intravenous lidocaine test was correlated with the subsequent response to mexiletine.[12]

The most common side-effects of lignocaine are neurological and include paresthesias, tremor, nausea, lightheadedness, hearing disturbances, slurred speech, and convulsions. Mexiletine is similarly associated with gastro-intestinal distress/nausea, dry mouth, and CNS symptoms including sleep disturbance, headaches, and drowsiness. Cardiac effects include bradycardia, hypotension, and arrhythmias. Patients with a history of myocardial dysfunction or arrhythmia may be at increased risk of serious cardiac events and should undergo an appropriate cardiac evaluation before local anaesthetic therapy is initiated. Given the increased risk of arrhythmias, tricyclic anti-depressants should be stopped at least 48 h before starting lignocaine or mexiletine.

A trial with an oral local anesthetic may be considered after anti-depressant and anti-convulsant drugs have been tried. Intravenous or subcutaneous lignocaine may be useful in the treatment of severe, rapidly increasing neuropathic pain.

Intravenous lignocaine usually is administered over 30 min: the dose ranges between 2 mg/kg and 5 mg/kg. Given the existence of a dose response curve, it is prudent to use a low dose infusion initially followed, if unsuccessful, by infusions at incrementally higher doses. If effective, the pain relief can continue for weeks. In patients with a frequent need of intravenous lignocaine infusions, a continuous subcutaneous infusion of 1–2 mg/kg/h lignocaine may be considered.

Treatment with mexiletine usually begins with a low dose (150 mg/day), which is followed by gradual dose escalation every 3–7 days to a maximum of 900–1200 mg/day.

NMDA receptor antagonists

Excitatory amino acids, such as glutamate and aspartate, are released by primary afferent neurons in response to noxious stimuli and are important in the central processing of the pain-related information. Interactions at the N-methyl-D-aspartate (NMDA) receptor are involved in the development of CNS changes that may underlie chronic pain and modulate opioid mechanisms—specifically tolerance. Pre-clinical studies have established that the N-methyl-D-aspartate receptor is involved in the sensitization of central neurones following injury and the development of the 'wind-up' phenomenon, a change in the response of central neurons that has been associated with neuropathic pain.

In the United States, the commercially available NMDA receptor antagonists include the dissociative anaesthetic ketamine, the antitussive dextromethorphan, and the antiviral amantadine. Each may be tried for neuropathic pain.

Some cancer patients with difficult neuropathic pain have experienced a substantial improvement in pain relief after the addition of ketamine to opioid therapy.

Ketamine can cause severe psychomimetic effects, however, such as nightmares and delirium, and the potential for this toxicity limits its use in the clinical setting. Haloperidol, diazepam, or midazolam are often co-administered to reduce the risk of these problems. Patients with intracranial hypertension or seizures should not receive this drug. There is some evidence that oral ketamine has a more favourable side-effect profile than parenteral ketamine, with drowsiness being the most common problem.[13] Oral ketamine can be added to the existing drug regimen in a dose of 0.5 mg/kg three times a day. An oral solution can be prepared by a pharmacy. In case of severe intractable neuropathic pain, ketamine can be given as continuous intravenous or subcutaneous infusion. It usually is initiated at a low dose (e.g. 1 mg/kg/h) and gradually increased.

Dextromethorphan has been found to be effective in the treatment of diabetic painful neuropathy and PHN. It may be initiated at a dose of 120–240 mg/day in three to four divided doses, and then increased gradually. Somnolence is a problem at higher doses. Experience with amantadine as an analgesic is very limited.

Other drug classes

Several other drug classes may be useful in the management of neuropathic pain (Table 9.4).

The GABA agonist baclofen has been shown to be effective in the treatment of trigeminal neuralgia and may be a useful drug for neuropathic pain in the medically ill. The most common side-effects are drowsiness, dizziness,

Table 9.4 Other oral adjuvant analgesics

Drug	Usually effective daily dose	Doses per day	Evidence
Local anaesthetics			
Mexiletine	150–900 mg	2–3	CT
NMDA antagonists			
Ketamine	1–5 mg/kg	2–3	OLT
Dextromethorphan	120–1000 mg	3–4	CT
Gaba agonist			
Baclofen	30–200 mg	2–3	CT
Benzodiazepines			
Alprazolam	0.75–1.5 mg	1–3	OLT
Diazepam	5–20 mg	1–3	CR

CT = controlled trials; OLT = open-label trials; CR = case report.

and gastro-intestinal distress. The incidence of these symptoms can be reduced by starting with a low dose (5–10 mg twice daily) and increasing it slowly. Baclofen cannot be discontinued abruptly after prolonged use, as hallucinations, manic psychotic episodes, or seizures may occur. Baclofen may be especially useful for patients with paroxysmal neuropathic pain.

Benzodiazepines also may have useful effects in patients with chronic cancer pain, and it may be impossible to determine the degree to which psychotropic or primary analgesic actions contribute to this outcome. The efficacy of clonazepam for neuropathic pain was noted previously and a survey of patients with mixed types of cancer-related neuropathic pains suggested that alprazolam also may have analgesic effects.[14] Patients with cancer pain commonly experience anxiety and muscle spasms, phenomena that may exacerbate the intensity of pain and respond well to other benzodiazepines, such as diazepam. Treatment should be started with the lowest possible dose (Table 9.4) and cognitive function must be monitored carefully during treatment.

Topical analgesic therapies

Recently, a lignocaine-impregnated patch (Lidoderm®) was approved for use in patients with PHN. This formulation appears to be well tolerated and should be considered for any patient who has a very localized neuropathic pain syndrome. Although the patch was studied with use limited to 12 h/day, continuous application is common in the clinical setting. Multiple patches are often used. There are limited data that indicate a high level of safety with up to three patches for periods up to 24 h. Application of more than three patches may be useful for some patients, but this approach should be accompanied by initial monitoring for local anaesthetic toxicity. An adequate trial may require several weeks of observation. The most frequently reported adverse event is mild to moderate skin redness, rash, or irritation at the patch.

Patients with localized neuropathic pain caused by peripheral nerve injury also can be considered for a trial of topical capsaicin, a peptide that depletes substance P in small primary afferent neurones. In a recent study in cancer patients with surgical neuropathic pain (e.g. post-mastectomy syndrome), capsaicin was found to significantly decrease pain and was preferred by 60% of the patients, despite side-effects such as skin burning.[15] Starting with the lower concentration formula (0.05%), and simultaneously using lidocaine 5% ointment or an oral analgesic, may help patients tolerate the initial burning discomfort. The burning frequently disappears over time with continuous use of three to four applications/day. Patients who do not see any improvement after one week are unlikely to benefit from further treatment.

Intra-spinal therapy and neural blockade

Another pharmacological strategy for the treatment of refractory neuropathic pain is neuraxial drug infusion. Given the high risk of epidural haematoma and possible neurological deficit due to compression of the spinal cord or nerve roots, placing an epidural catheter is contra-indicated in patients with platelet counts below 50 000/μl.

Neuropathic pain may be as poorly responsive to spinal opioids alone as it is to systemic opioids, and the co-administration of a local anaesthetic or alpha-2-adrenergic agonists (e.g. clonidine) may provide additional analgesia and permit the successful treatment of patients unresponsive to spinal morphine alone. In an uncontrolled study in patients with severe refractory cancer pain, a constant intrathecal infusion of 0.5 mg/ml morphine, plus 4.75 mg/ml bupivacaine, resulted in good pain relief in all 53 patients. The most common side-effects were urinary retention, paresthesias, and paresis/gait impairment, which occurred in approximately one-third of the patients.[16] In another study, the epidural infusion of bupivacaine 0.1–0.5%, in addition to morphine, also was highly efficacious.[17] Sensory loss was consistently observed only at bupivacaine concentrations exceeding 0.25%, and motor impairment occurred only at concentrations exceeding 0.35%. In a controlled study in 85 cancer patients with refractory pain syndromes, 30 μg/h epidural clonidine, together with rescue epidural morphine, provided good pain relief in 56% of patients with neuropathic pain.[18] The most common side-effects of intra-spinal clonidine are hypotension and bradycardia, and patients should be monitored thoroughly during the first days treatment.

In a large controlled trial in patients with poorly opioid responsive pain, the continuous intra-thecal drug application via an implantable drug delivery system plus comprehensive medical management resulted in better pain control, less fatigue and improved survival than comprehensive medical management alone.[19]

There is good evidence that invasive techniques such as local anaesthetic peripheral and sympathetic nerve blocks, and neurolytic blocks may reduce analgesic requirements in poorly-responsive neuropathic pain syndromes. Given the risk of exacerbating pain and serious complications, they have to be considered carefully and only after the pain syndrome has been shown to be refractory to several trials of adjuvant drugs. However, nerve blocks may be particularly helpful in patients suffering from incident neuropathic pain. Prior to attempting pain relief through neurolytic blockade, a prognostic block using a local anaesthetic may be of help to predict the degree of pain relief and potential complications associated with the respective neurolytic block.

Conclusion

The treatment of neuropathic pain that is poorly responsive to opioids can be a challenging problem in patients with haematological malignancies. The pharmacological options available for neuropathic pain have, however, advanced rapidly in recent years and clinical experience suggests that most patients can be managed by the addition of an adjuvant analgesic. After a comprehensive assessment, clinicians should be able to choose among the diverse range of treatment options available and implement an approach, or combination of approaches, that will have a high probability of improving pain relief in their patients.

References

1 Bauduer, F., Capdupuy, C., and Renoux, M. (2000). Characteristics of death in a department of oncohaematology within a general hospital. A study of 81 cases. *Support Care Cancer* **8**, 302–306.

2 McGrath, P. (2002). Qualitative findings on the experience of end-of-life care for haematological malignancies. *Am J Hosp Pall Care* **19**, 103–111, 2002.

3 Portenoy, R. K., Foley, K. M., and Inturrisi, C. E. (1990). The nature of opioid responsiveness and its implications for neuropathic pain: New hypotheses derived from studies of opioid infusions. *Pain* **43**, 273–286.

4 Quasthoff, S. and Hartung, H. P. (2002). Chemotherapy-induced peripheral neuropathy. *J Neurol* **249**, 9–17.

5 Mercadante, S. and Portenoy, R. K. (2001). Opioid poorly-responsive cancer pain. Part 3: Clinical strategies to improve opioid responsiveness. *J Pain Symptom Manage* **21**, 338–354.

6 Backonja, M., Beydoun, A., Edwards, K. R. *et al.* (1998). Gabapentin for the symptomatic treatment of painful neuropathy in patients with diabetes mellitus: a randomized controlled trial. *JAMA* **280**, 1831–1836.

7 Rowbotham, M., Harden, N., Stacey, B. *et al.* (1998). Gabapentin for the treatment of postherpetic neuralgia: a randomized controlled trial. *JAMA* **280**, 1837–1842.

8 Caraceni, A., Zecca, E., Martini, C. *et al.* (1999). Gabapentin as an adjuvant to opioid analgesia for neuropathic cancer pain. *J Pain and Symptom Manage* **17**, 441–445.

9 Morello, C. M., Lechband, S. G., Stoner, C. P. *et al.* (1999). Randomized double blind trial of gabapentin with amitryptiline in diabetic peripheral neuropathy pain. *Arch Intern Med* **59**, 1931–1937.

10 Eija, K., Tiina, T., and Neuvonen Pertti, J. (1995). Amitriptyline effectively relieves neuropathic pain following treatment of breast cancer. *Pain* **64**, 293–302.

11 Chong, S. F., Bretscher, M. E., Mailliard, J. A. *et al.* (1997). Pilot study evaluating local anesthetics administered systemically for treatment of pain in patients with advanced cancer. *J Pain Symptom Manage* **13**, 112–117.

12 Galer, B. S., Harle, J., and Rowbotham, M. C. (1996). Response to intravenous lidocaine infusion predicts subsequent response to oral mexiletine: a prospective study. *J Pain Symptom Manage* **12**, 161–167.

13 Thogulava, R. K., Saxena, A., Bhatnagar, S. *et al.* (2002). Oral ketamine as an adjuvant to oral morphine for neuropathic pain in cancer patients. *J Pain Symptom Manage* 23, 60–65.

14 Fernandez, F., Adams, F., and Holmes, V. F. (1987). Analgesic effect of alprazolam in patients with chronic, organic pain of malignant origin. *J Clin Psychopharmacol* 7,167–169.

15 Ellison, N., Loprinzi, C. L., Kugler, J. *et al.* (1997). Phase III placebo-controlled trial of capsaicin cream in the management of surgical neuropathic pain in cancer patients. *J Clin Oncol* 15, 2974–2980.

16 Sjoberg, M., Nitescu, P., Appelgren, L. *et al.* (1994). Long-term intrathecal morphine and bupivacaine in patients with refractory cancer pain. Results from a morphine: bupivacaine dose regimen of 0.5:4.75 mg/ml. *Anesthesiology* 80, 284–297.

17 Du Pen, S. L., Kharash, E. D., Williams, A. *et al.* (1992). Chronic epidural bupivacaine-opioid infusion in intractable cancer pain. *Pain* 49, 293–300.

18 Eisenach, J. C., DuOen, S., Dubois, M. *et al.* (1995). Epidural clonidine analgesia for intractable cancer pain. The epidural clonidine study group. *Pain* 61, 391–399.

19 Smith, T. J., Staats, P., Deer, T. *et al.* (2002). Randomized clinical trial of an implantable drug delivery system compared with comprehensive medical management for refractory cancer pain: impact on pain, drug-related toxicity, and survival. *J Clin Oncol* 20, 4040–9.

Chapter 10

Changing the emphasis from active curative care to active palliative care in haematology patients

David Jeffrey and Ray Owen

Introduction

Almost all transitions are psychologically challenging for those involved. The transition between a curative and a palliative approach to the care of a patient with a haematological malignancy may present challenges for patients, families, and healthcare professionals. This chapter identifies these challenges, illustrating them with clinical scenarios, and explores the reasons why the situations are difficult. Finally, ways of improving the situation are suggested. Many of these problems at the interface between curative and palliative care are complex, and we provide frameworks to stimulate thought and discussion, rather than definitive solutions.

What is the difference between 'active curative' and 'active palliative'?

The care of a patient with cancer is often likened to a 'journey', which may be conveniently divided into stages. Each stage is defined by the primary aim of treatment and care: curative, palliative, and terminal.[1] However, in a clinical setting the boundaries between these stages are not clearly defined.[2]

Defining the stages of cancer care

Curative In this phase of care there is a realistic chance of cure or of long-lasting remission. The aim of treatment is survival of the patient. Some harmful side-effects of treatment may be acceptable to the patient in the hope of cure.[3] However, the patient and doctor may have a different understanding of the term 'cure'. The patient may expect more than survival and be hoping for a return to the normality that existed before the onset of the disease.[3] On the other hand, doctors may measure cure in terms of 5-year disease-free survival.

Palliative Palliative care has been defined by the World Health Organization (WHO)[4]:

> Palliative care is the active total care of patients whose disease is not responsive to curative treatment. Control of pain, of other symptoms and of psychological, social and spiritual problems is paramount. The goal of palliative care is achievement of the best quality of life for patients and their families. Many aspects of palliative care are also applicable earlier in the course of the illness, in conjunction with anticancer treatment.

Palliative care thus:

♦ affirms life and regards dying as a normal process

♦ neither hastens or postpones death

♦ provides relief from pain and other symptoms

♦ integrates the psychological and spiritual aspects of patient care

♦ offers a support system to help patients live as actively as possible until death

♦ offers a support system to help the family cope during the patient's illness and in their own environment.[4]

This definition now needs clarification. 'Total care', in the definition, refers to the holistic approach to the care of the patient. It does not mean that specialist palliative care services should take over the total care of the patient. Specialist palliative care services act as a resource to the primary professional carers. Furthermore, it may not be possible to 'control' psychological, social, or spiritual problems, as the definition seems to suggest. It is crucial, however, that these dimensions of care are assessed and addressed as far as possible.

The statement 'neither hastens or postpones death' reflects the philosophy of palliative care, which rejects active euthanasia as a means of relieving suffering.[5] Palliative treatments may lengthen survival, but this is not their primary goal, which is to improve quality of life. Palliative care involves more than the control of symptoms, it aims to relieve suffering, a more subtle concept that embraces the ways in which the illness affects the individual. In the palliative phase there is a shift in emphases from quantity of life to quality of life and from pathology to person.[6]

Terminal In this phase the aim of care is to enable the patient to die with dignity. Harmful or distressing side-effects of treatment are not acceptable.[1]

The nature of the challenges at the transition

At transitions, uncertainties exist for patients and their families, and for the healthcare professionals looking after them. Clinicians may be caught in a dilemma between over-treating patients on the one hand or neglecting a remote chance of cure on the other. Death and dying may be perceived as failures of an ever more sophisticated medical technology, rather than an appropriate and natural consequence of potentially lethal diseases. Predicting when death is going to occur is difficult. Often patients or their families may try to persuade doctors to continue with curative attempts even when the doctor has suggested that they are no longer beneficial.[7] The timing of the change from a curative to a palliative approach to caring, presents clinical and moral challenges, which are now discussed.

Challenges for healthcare professionals

When does palliative care begin?

Calman argues that palliative care begins when 'the diagnosis of cancer is established, death is certain and likely in the near future, and a curative approach to care has been abandoned'.[8] However, this definition does not help us to decide when the curative approach should be abandoned.

Challenge: When does palliative care begin?

Example: The patient says, 'I'm not bad enough for palliative care, am I?'.

Why is it a problem?

- The haematologist may still have some options for active care. Because an option for treatment exists does not mean that it must be used.
- The haematologist may feel a sense of failure, or guilt for abandoning the patient.
- The haematologist may be concerned that the mention of palliative care will be too distressing for the patient or destroy all hope.
- The patient/family may demand further treatment directed against the disease.
- The patient/professionals may equate palliative care with terminal care.
- The patient may be denied the broader input offered by specialist palliative care if referral does not take place, with a reduction in quality of life.
- The patient may fear that this forces them to confront issues (including with family) that they do not feel ready for yet.

Challenge: When does palliative care begin? *(continued)*

How to address the challenge?

- Making sure that specialist palliative care is introduced early enough in the illness trajectory.
- Clear referral criteria for specialist palliative care should be available.
- Using specialist palliative care teams frequently enough for everyone (including patients) to be familiar with their role.
- Identifying and addressing the patient's fears about palliative care and its implications.
- Once the patient meets the specialist palliative care team member, they should negotiate the nature of their future involvement.

Multiprofessional teamworking

The physical, social, psychological, spiritual, and emotional needs of the patient and their family are complex and are beyond the skills of any individual professional. Multiprofessional teamworking is an essential element of modern healthcare and offers both potential benefits and harms for patients. A detailed account of the dynamics of teamwork is beyond the scope of this chapter. Haematologists involved in the curative phases of a patient's care often develop close relationships with the patient and family, and may even act as a surrogate general practitioner. In such a context it may be difficult to involve another specialist team.

Challenge: Referring to another professional team

Example: Consultant haematologist says, 'I know about treating bone pain—why do we need specialist palliative care involvement?'.

Why is it a problem?

- Problems may extend beyond the symptom: anxieties/concerns, social/financial difficulties, problems at home, and the haematology team may not have:
  - time to assess fully
  - access to an extended support network to address these issues.
- Patient may downplay symptoms to 'protect' the doctor who has been trying to effect a cure.

Challenge: Referring to another professional team *(continued)*

◆ Without realizing it, the doctor may be acting on basis of concern for professional boundaries, rather than optimal teamwork.

◆ Asking for external help may seem like an admission of failure.

How to address the challenge?

◆ Developing good working relationship and trust over time (rather than just dealing with isolated cases).

◆ Joint discussion of *potential* referrals between haematology and palliative care teams.

◆ Multidisciplinary team (MDT) meetings.

◆ Early referral to specialist palliative care.

◆ Allow the patient time to adjust to changes in goals of care.

◆ Raise awareness of availability of palliative care in curative phase, e.g. written information.

Communication

A patient needs to have information about the diagnosis, prognosis, treatment options and side-effects and sources of support if he/she is to be able to make realistic choices. Communication involves both giving information and listening to the concerns of the patient and family. Good communication is necessary:

◆ to maintain trust

◆ to reduce uncertainty

◆ to prevent unrealistic expectations

◆ to allow the patient to adjust

◆ to prevent a conspiracy of silence.[9]

There are a number of barriers which present challenges to good communication.

Privacy

We owe patients a duty of confidentiality, but in practice this duty is often breached.

Time

A partnership between the patient and doctor means that the two parties are working towards a common goal. Doctors, while experts in the areas of diagnosis

Challenge: Privacy

Example: May need to tell the bed-bound patient, with their partner, on a full hospital ward, that cure is no longer an option.

Why is it a problem?

• Loss of confidentiality.

• May inhibit questions asked/answered.

• May inhibit expression of emotion.

• May traumatize other patients/relatives.

How to address the challenge?

• Plan ahead, try to arrange for some private space to be available.

• Use other spaces, even if you have to wheel the bed there (setting this up can act as a 'warning shot'; e.g. 'We've got some important things to discuss, so I'd like us to have a bit of privacy...').

• Consider moving others out if necessary and feasible.

• Advocate for interview rooms as essential equipment for a ward.

and treatment options, do not have sufficient expertise in patients' social, psychological, or spiritual attitudes, beliefs, and values to be able to make choices for them.[10] Patients vary in the extent to which they wish to be involved in decision-making. The same patient may express different choices to different members of the multidisciplinary team, or vary his/her choices from time to time. The key to unravelling this complex situation is to give the patient time and not to make assumptions. In the general practice setting, the patient's feeling of empowerment to make decisions and choices has been shown to be related to consultation length.[11]

Challenge: Spending time to listen to the patient's concerns

Example: Thinks haematologist, 'I am an hour behind in this outpatient clinic, I will have to catch up'.

Why is it a problem?

• Workload pressures.

• Doctors are perceived by patients to be busy.

Challenge: Spending time to listen to the patient's concerns *(continued)*

- Non-verbal cues that doctor is harassed.
- Patient does not want to keep others waiting even longer.
- Patients need time to reflect on information.
- Managerial focus on 20-minute wait.
- It may be quicker to prescribe treatment than to explore the patient's concerns.
- Communication with team members and with general practitioners takes a great deal of time.

How to address the challenge?

- Need to value time spent listening as 'doing something'.
- Adequate resourcing and manageable workloads for haematologists and the team.
- Using the whole team, specialist nurses or the palliative care team may be able to give more time.
- Realistic time-management in planning of clinics and ward rounds.
- Improve the healthcare professionals' communication skills by suitable advanced training.
- Develop clear lines of communication between primary and secondary care.
- Remember that time taken avoiding misunderstandings and conflict is less than the time taken resolving them.

Who else to have present?

Challenge: Who else to have present

Example: On a busy ward round with a nurse, registrar, and two medical students, a patient with advanced lymphoma asks, 'Am I going to get better?'. The patient's wife has, in the past, attended all his out-patient clinic appointments with him and she is not on the ward at present.

Why is it a problem?

- Confidentiality.
- Lack of privacy.

Challenge: Who else to have present *(continued)*

◆ No relatives present.

◆ Too many people around the patient.

◆ Not everyone wants a partner present; the patient may have been desperate for the chance to catch you alone.

How to address the challenge?

◆ Try to ensure privacy.

◆ Ask the patient who he/she would like to be present, e.g. 'That's clearly an important conversation—would you prefer to have it when your wife can be present?'.

◆ Make sure you have time.

◆ Anticipate the difficult question.

◆ Have the appropriate factual information at hand.

Prognostic uncertainty

This uncertainty creates communication problems for patients, their families, and the professionals. Patients and families often need information to gain a sense of control of their situation and to make plans, and doctors are conscious of the difficulties inherent in trying to estimate a prognosis for an individual.

Challenge: Estimating a patient's prognosis

Example: A patient with relapsed non-Hodgkin's lymphoma asks, 'How long have I got?'.

Why is it a problem?

◆ Impossible to be certain what will happen to an individual.

◆ Doctors and nurses are often wrong in their estimates of survival time.

◆ Fear of distressing the patient.

◆ Memories of an individual patient in the past who did surprisingly well.

◆ Sometimes a patient may ask impulsively without thinking through whether they really want to know.

How to address the challenge?

◆ Try to find out what the patient thinks—check that he/she does really want to know.

Challenge: Estimating a patient's prognosis *(continued)*

- Tailor the information to the needs of the patient—the patient may simply want to know that it will not be today or tomorrow, and benefit from reassurance that there will be a warning when the time gets nearer.
- What is behind the question?
- Acknowledge the uncertainty.
- Set realistic goals.
- Discuss unfinished business.
- May need to discuss fears of death and dying.

Talking about death and dying

There is a feeling in society that talking about death and dying is morbid, and a fear exists for some that talking about it can bring it about. This can be a reason why many healthy adults are reluctant to make a will.

Challenge: Talking about death and dying

Example: A patient with advanced myeloma with marrow failure asks, 'Will there be terrible pain at the end?'.

Why is it a problem?

- Doctors and nurses have their own fears.
- Death and dying may be viewed as medical failure.
- Society still views these as taboo subjects.
- Fear that talking about it may bring it about.
- Genuine uncertainty about what will happen to the individual.
- Issue is often left until the patient is weak and exhausted.
- Staff/relatives may view 'fear of death' as the complete explanation for the patient's distress, rather than exploring what they fear most about death, e.g. Will I die alone? Who will look after my children?

How to address the challenge?

- Be accessible and ask open questions that encourage patients to raise these issues, if they wish.
- Acknowledge uncertainty.
- Continuity of care.
- Training for staff in communication skills.
- Use the team.

Ethical issues: withholding and withdrawing life-prolonging medical treatments

One of the changes at the interface between curative and palliative care is a change in emphasis in the aim of care from quantity of life to quality of life. Staff may be involved in stopping further blood transfusions, discontinuing antibiotics, or stopping further chemotherapy. Each management decision should be tailored to the individual and any decision of this kind must protect the dignity, comfort, and rights of the patient, and take into account the patient's wishes.[12] Advances in medical technology extend treatment options and general guidance is offered here as a framework to aid decision-making.

Do not attempt resuscitation decisions

Talking about 'Do not attempt resuscitation decisions' is difficult for many doctors. Doctors need to be able to discuss with patients that a treatment is not appropriate, when it is unlikely to confer benefit or when it is likely to cause more harm than good. Refusing a treatment may be difficult for doctors, particularly when it may appear that a 'life is at stake'. However, in patients dying with advanced cancer, attempting cardio-pulmonary resuscitation (CPR) promotes the myth that doctors can postpone death indefinitely.[13]

Challenge: Talking about do not attempt resuscitation decisions

Example: The patient refuses a DNAR decision by the haematology team.

Why is it a problem?

- Doctors may lack communication skills.
- Fear of litigation.
- Sense of failure.
- Fear of causing distress to patient and family.
- Who should discuss?
- Poor inter-professional communication may lead to lack of consensus within the team.
- Guidelines are contradictory.[14]
- Patient and relatives lack knowledge of the process involved and that it does not necessarily work.
- Patients may think that agreeing to a DNAR order, is to give up.

Challenge: Talking about do not attempt resuscitation decisions *(continued)*

- Discussion often postponed until patient is too ill to participate.
- Even if the hospital team, patient, and family agree on a DNAR order, others may need to be aware; e.g. the crew of the ambulance taking the patient home on discharge.

How to address the challenge?

- Patients need better education on CPR outcomes.
- Respect for autonomy restricts CPR use when it is refused by a patient but cannot create a 'right to CPR'.
- Locally agreed policies on CPR and DNAR decisions are necessary, these should include ambulance services.
- Communication about DNAR decisions should take place as part of a wider discussion of treatment goals at an earlier stage in the patient's illness.
- DNAR decisions should be recorded in the notes in the appropriate manner and discussed with the nursing team—involve palliative care team in problematic cases.

Stopping palliative chemotherapy

Challenge: Stopping palliative chemotherapy

Example: A patient with chemo-resistant lymphoma, for whom further therapy would be futile asks, 'So what will you do now doctor?'.

Why is it a problem?

- Doctors do not want to appear to have 'given up' on a patient.
- Legal uncertainty.
- Patient may equate palliative care referral with imminent death.
- Patient may feel that there is a question of best use of resources and that they are being denied treatment on financial grounds.

How to address the challenge?

- Good communication with patient's family and the rest of the professional team.
- Investigating all possibilities.

Challenge: Stopping palliative chemotherapy *(continued)*

♦ Ensuring that palliative chemotherapy is improving the patient's quality of life by monitoring the patient's view during therapy.

♦ Primary goal of medicine is to benefit the patient.

♦ Treatment that does not provide net benefit to the patient may be ethically and legally, withheld or withdrawn, and the goal of care should shift to palliation of symptoms.

Emotional strain

Any healthcare environment can be stressful. In addition to the usual workload-related factors, emotional strain can be caused by working closely with people who are suffering, in distress, and sometimes facing a poor prognosis. Haematology units tend to attract dedicated staff who work hard to encourage and support patients through often difficult treatment regimens during the curative phase. These staff form a close emotional bond with the patient and family, and share some of their distress when the disease relapses and prolonged survival is no longer possible. Sometimes death follows quickly after chemotherapy has been discontinued; patients are often young with dependent children and staff may well become emotionally involved in the patient's struggle, and eventual death.

Emotional bonds

Challenge: Close bonds can arise between staff and patients—when the outlook is bleak for the patient, it can impact on the staff

Example: You have been closely supporting a patient with a young family, who then finds out that cure is no longer possible.

Why is it a problem?

♦ Effective care may mean you have got to know the person well.

♦ There will always be some patients/families you identify with yourself/your own.

♦ Their helplessness may transfer to you.

♦ It can be harder to cope with deaths if there was a reasonable chance of cure initially, than if the condition was palliative from diagnosis.

Challenge: Close bonds can arise between staff and patients—when the outlook is bleak for the patient, it can impact on the staff *(continued)*

How to address the challenge?

◆ Stay aware of boundaries, and question if you find yourself thinking about a specific patient/family much of the time.

◆ If you think you (or a colleague) are getting too close, try to 'share the care' with other team members.

◆ Know where you get your support from (Colleagues? Formal team meetings? Formal supervision?) and make use of it.

◆ Remember that if we *never* feel involved, and we *never* feel sad, then it is probably time to find a different job.

Grieving

Challenge: Grief for patients

Example: A well-known patient finally dies.

Why is it a problem?

◆ Distressing.

◆ Can intrude into personal life.

◆ May feel it impairs our dealings with the relatives who are 'really' grieving, or undermines our professionalism, if visibly upset.

How to address this challenge?

◆ Allow ourselves to be sad sometimes.

◆ Accept that signs of our upset (providing not excessive) can be appreciated by relatives.

◆ Use support networks (as described above).

◆ If several staff are affected by a particular death, consider having a defuse/debrief session, possibly facilitated by someone external to, but trusted by, the team.

Challenges for the patient and family

The change from active curative to active palliative will change the patient and family's world-view, and indeed their world. Every patient, every family, and every individual within a family, will respond to this differently—we can never predict how. These differences in reaction arise mainly from different understanding and different thoughts regarding the situation:

> We do not react to events, but to the view we take of them.
> Epictetus, *The Discourses*

Whilst the individual responses will differ, many of our patients moving from curative to palliative care, will face characteristic changes, challenges, and problems.:

How do people make sense of illness?

After study of lay 'commonsense' models of illness, Leventhal identified that most people trying to understand an illness seek information in the following areas[15]:

♦ **Identity:** What's it called? What are its symptoms?

♦ **Cause:** How did I come to have it?

♦ **Consequences:** How will it affect me? How will it affect those around me?

♦ **Timeline:** How will it change over time (e.g. resolving, chronic, remitting/relapsing, deteriorating).

♦ **Cure/Control:** Can it be cured? How? If not, can it be controlled? How?

If we imagine Mr X moving from active curative treatment to palliative treatment, we can see that all of these (with possible exception of cause) will change (Table 10.1).

Understanding the treatment choices

We know that patients view palliative treatments, and their worth, differently from most healthcare staff; they appearing willing to undergo more aversive treatment for less chance of benefit and less longevity of benefit than most staff would consider worthwhile.[7]

The theory of planned behaviour is one of the standard models of how people make any sort of planned action (in this case, undertake a specific treatment).[16] It identifies the main factors shaping attitude to an action as being:

1. What are the costs and benefits of this course of action?

2. What do others (who matter to me) think about this?

3. Will I be able to do it?

If we imagine a patient moving from curative to palliative care, we can see that all of these may change (Table 10.2).

Table 10.1 How do people make sense of illness

	Before transition	After transition
Identity	Non-Hodgkins lymphoma (NHL)	Chemo-resistant high grade NHL
Cause	Do not know	Do not know
Consequences	It makes me very weak, unable to work, or to fulfill family expectations. Very hard to get out of house.	Now it is making me even weaker. I am unable to care for myself. I can now do very few physical things, though I am still mostly alert and mentally competent.
Timeline	I will be really ill for a while, but should then recover and return to normal.	I am not going to recover. I will probably die within the next few weeks/months.
Cure control	With aggressive treatment (which may be physically unpleasant and require isolation) the condition should be cured.	It cannot be cured. The disease itself cannot be controlled, but symptoms such as pain and nausea should be.

Note that if Mr X's 'representation' of his illness remains unchanged, despite the change in prognosis. He may make decisions with regard to treatment, he may communicate with family members and make personal arrangements, which seem inappropriate; this may cause problems.

Challenge: Understand the illness

Example: A patient's wife cannot understand why you were hoping for 'cure' a few days ago, but now are talking about palliative care.

Why a problem?
Misunderstandings can lead to:

◆ lack of informed consent
◆ resentment and complaints
◆ apparently irrational behaviour
◆ helplessness/dependency.

How to address the challenge?

◆ Make use of other team members to reinforce explanations.
◆ Give access to written materials, BACUP booklets, websites, etc.
◆ Ask patient to explain to *you* what they understand of their condition.
◆ Assess their understanding, and fit your information to common lay information needs.
◆ Remember not everyone wants *all* the information at once—ask how much they want.

Table 10.2 How do people choose treatments?

	Curative approach	Palliative approach
Costs vs. benefits	The side-effects may be awful, but its worth putting up with them to get my old life back.	There does not seem to be many side-effects, but it will be hard to start a treatment that I know will not cure me.
What do others think?	Everyone thinks I should do this—the doctors seem optimistic, and my husband thinks we should try anything to get me better.	The doctor seemed a bit sad when he told me; perhaps he does not approve of giving up. And my husband thinks they should still be trying to cure me.
Will I be able to do it?	I am worried that I will not be able to cope with the nausea, the fatigue, and being confined to the unit.	I think this sounds a lot easier to bear than some of the treatments I had in the past.

Similar factors will be influencing how a *relative* perceives a given action/treatment plan.

Challenge: Understanding the treatment choices

Example: Patient seeks curative treatments, even though in the team's opinion palliative approaches are more appropriate.

Why is it a problem?

♦ May lead to tension between team and patient/family, especially if requested treatments cannot be provided.

♦ Patient may have treatment-related reduction in quality of life in final weeks without any survival gain.

♦ Missed opportunities for patient and family preparation for death (communication, making arrangements, seeing relatives, etc.).

♦ 'Driving force' for this approach may not come from patient, but rather from other family member who has not yet accepted situation.

How to address the challenge?

♦ Try to establish patient and family's perception of the situation— preferably in separate interviews (as in a joint interview they may distort their views to 'protect' others present).

Challenge: Understanding the treatment choices *(continued)*

- Identify factors shaping treatment choice (see text above for common factors), especially what significant others think.
- Acknowledge the costs as well as the benefits of the treatments under consideration.

Relationships

Maintaining key relationships is one of the most important tasks in coping with major life changes.

With family

Challenge: May not be open communication between family members

Example: Patient may not want to tell family that cure is no longer possible.

Why is it a problem?

- Family may push for inappropriate treatments.
- May become angry at team for 'giving up' on patient.
- Patient may feel isolated as they cannot confide in family members.
- Lack of opportunity to discuss important issues, make arrangements, make wishes known (terminal decline may be too rapid to correct this situation).
- May make grieving process more problematic for surviving family.

How to address the challenge?

- Explore reasons for reluctance to communicate.
- If fear is for psychological impact of news on family, discuss support available professionally, and identify existing support networks in family/community.
- Help patient see the potential costs, not just the perceived benefits, of collusion.
- If helpful (and patient agrees), offer to meet jointly with patient and partner, and break the bad news yourself.
- Remember, the patients relationship with their family is more important, and has a longer history, than their relationship with you; how they choose to handle things may be very different to how you would.

With professionals

> ### Challenge: Patients may have developed great faith in their healthcare team, and may sometimes feel let down when cure fails
>
> Example: Patient says to doctor, 'You're the one who persuaded me to go through all that awful treatment—how can you now tell me I'm going to die anyway?'.
>
> Why is it a problem?
>
> + Being a patient always involves some reliance on a healthcare team.
> + You may have needed to strongly emphasize optimism with a patient, especially if they have been emotionally low; this optimism can in retrospect seem unrealistic.
> + If the patient *perceives* that promises did not come true, they may not believe reassurances about palliative interventions.
> + The staff member may also feel some sense of failure (see 'emotional bonds' above).
>
> How to address the challenge?
>
> + Allow expression of thoughts and feelings on the subject.
> + Without being 'defensive', gently remind the patient why they undertook treatment, why it was worthwhile trying, even though success was *never* guaranteed.
> + Express your own regret that treatment did not work, without giving the false impression that you personally failed (which would be unhelpful for everyone).
> + Emphasize that you are not 'giving up' on them, hence active palliative approach.

Quality of Life

Like many others, this is a term more frequently cited than adequately defined. At heart, it refers to the importance of psychological, social, and functional state. The key determinant is not the absolute level of these states, but the degree of match/mismatch with that person's expectations. Using Calman's model of quality of life, the greater the 'gap' between a patient's expectations and the reality of their situation, the poorer their quality of life.[17] Sometimes, our role is as much to modify expectations as to modify state.

Two areas that can prove problematic are questions of 'hope' and whether this is 'a life worth living'.

Hope

Challenge: Realizing that cure is no longer possible can be perceived as removing all hope

Example: Patient says, 'They've told me they can't cure me—there's no hope left for me now'.

Why is it a problem?

- While cure still appears possible, most people pin their hopes on that, and may not realize that there are other things to hope for.
- Hopelessness is a major factor in the development of significant depression and the desire to die.
- Patient may not 'see the point' in any interventions (including palliative ones).
- Patient's hopelessness can be very distressing for family members.

How to address the challenge?

- Acknowledge their sadness and the difficulty of finding no cure after they have fought so hard.
- Emphasize that there are other things to hope for—comfort, good symptom control, seeing their family, etc.
- Develop some realistic aims and plans for them to work towards.
- Be alert for development of depression (see below).

A life worth living

Many people with serious illnesses (or without) may end up wondering 'what's the point of carrying on?'. In conditions with rapid progress from health, to acute illness, then curative treatment, then palliative care, the speed of transition may overwhelm mechanisms of psychological adjustment (which are not infallible in themselves). When in active curative treatment, people may sustain themselves by dreaming of a return to their previous life (or indeed an idealized version of it); when it becomes clear that this will never happen, the patient may not consider any existence to be worth living.

Challenge: Even with good palliative care, the patient may not consider what is on offer is 'a life worth living'

Example: Patient says, 'It's not worth carrying on like this—I may as well die now'.

Why is it a problem?

◆ Such thoughts lead to emotions of sadness and misery.

◆ Can lead to suicidal tendencies, or requests for euthanasia.

◆ Can lead to reduced activity, withdrawal from contact with others, intensifying a downward spiral into depression.

How to address the challenge?

◆ Acknowledge the losses and the suddenness of change.

◆ After the initial shock has passed, try to establish what things now matter most to them (e.g. time with family, helping their children, enjoying the garden); find out what activities may supply these qualities within the realm of what is possible (e.g. a drive to an accessible beauty spot, as climbing a mountain is no longer possible).

◆ Some things (listening to music, watching a movie) may still be possible, but warn that they 'might not feel the same' at first.

Emotional responses

Many expectations of how patients react have been shaped by models such as that of Kubler-Ross[18] (or often, by simplifications and distortions of such models), which suggest that certain sequences of emotional reaction are more common than others. In reality, it seems that almost any emotional reaction can occur at any time, and not necessarily only one at a time! Here, we discuss three common emotional responses at this transition point.

Anger

Challenge: Patient may experience, and possibly express, anger

Example: Patient appears shorter-tempered generally, then one day shouts, 'If you doctors actually listened to your patients, maybe this cancer would have been caught in time'.

Challenge: Patient may experience, and possibly express, anger *(continued)*

Why is it a problem?

- Can take varied forms—related to a single issue, to multiple issues, or generally irritability.
- Sustained arousal and rumination can sap energy and create physical discomfort.
- Can distance patient from family and friends.
- Can interfere with trust of healthcare team.
- Can lead to defensiveness and/or demoralization of treatment team.

How to address the challenge?

- Acknowledge anger and (where possible) demonstrate that you have grasped what they are angry about.
- Do not 'dismiss' the anger as part of adjustment, but suggest that things seem even worse to someone facing that.
- Identify if there is anything that the patient or family should/can do to address the source of their anger.
- If anger persists, try to get the patient to see that, no matter how *justified* the anger is, it is beginning to affect them adversely.
- If they agree, think about simple anger-management techniques (relaxation training, distraction activities, limiting rumination/mental rehearsal of problems and arguments); seek advice from psychology or psychiatry services if necessary.

Depression

Some degree of sadness may be inevitable in these circumstances; major depression is not. It is impossible to be confident about the incidence of depression in a population like this; rates depend entirely upon the detail of criteria used, and are confused further by the effects of the illness. The common assumption that depression is under-reported and under-treated in palliative populations is, however, probably a fair one.

Challenge: Patient/relative may become depressed

Example: Patient becomes uncharacteristically tearful, withdrawn and apathetic and stays that way for a fortnight.

Challenge: Patient/relative may become depressed *(continued)*

Why is it a problem?

- Depression is a distressing and debilitating state. It is not the way most people would choose to spend a limited life-expectancy.
- It interferes with family relationships, causing wider distress.
- It may mask/mimic/interact with disease-related symptoms (fatigue, anorexia, decreased sex-drive), making management harder.
- It can lead to reduced activity, decreased pleasurable events, and increased rumination, causing further lowering of mood, thereby creating a 'vicious circle'.

How to address the challenge?

- Assess carefully: as 'biological signs' may be unhelpful, look for anhedonia (inability to experience pleasure, even when 'positive' things are happening), global hopelessness, or novel low self-worth.
- Encourage activity and distraction.
- Provide supportive counselling.
- If it does not improve, consider anti-depressant medication and referral to clinical psychology/liaison psychiatry, if available.

Anxiety

Like sadness, some degree of anxiety may be inevitable. However, it can intensify into a significant anxiety problem; one of the more common forms of this, at transition to palliative care, is panic attacks.

Challenge: Development of panic attacks

Example: In days after being told that the condition is no longer curable, the patient reports episodes of sudden-onset breathlessness, tachycardia, palpitations, dizziness, and is convinced that s/he is dying.

Why is it a problem?

- For physiological anxiety symptoms to escalate into a panic attack, the patient usually has to have a catastrophic interpretation of them; transition to palliative care makes it easy to think, 'I'm dying'.

Challenge: Development of panic attacks *(continued)*

- Can become self-sustaining; even if the patient realizes that they are not imminently dying, the experience is so unpleasant that the thought, 'I'm going to have a panic attack' can be catastrophic enough to escalate the attack.
- It may mask/mimic/interact with disease-related symptoms, making management harder.
- It can be very distressing for the family to see.

How to address the challenge?

- As far as possible, exclude organic bases of symptoms (e.g. lung problems). Please note: even if there are organic components of presentation, there may still be a panic reaction to them, and panic-management techniques may still be helpful (see below).
- Ask, 'What goes through your mind when you're feeling like this?'; the patient may have misconceptions that simple information will clear up.
- Discuss with the patient the difference between normal worry and panic.
- If relevant, discuss the difference between thinking, 'I will die in few months', as opposed to, 'These feelings mean I'm dying at this instant'.
- Treatment of choice is a cognitive-behavioural approach, involving challenging catastrophic thoughts, breathing control, and relaxation. If no-one on the team is able to deliver this, consider referral to psychology/psychiatry, or some physiotherapy departments.
- If the patient is unable to approach the problem in this way (e.g. too ill, too confused), then consider medication-based approach.

Conclusion

There may have been a time when the end of curative treatment did mean, 'There's nothing more we can do for you'. Fortunately, there is now a great deal that can be done for people reaching this stage of their disease. But to deliver this care in an effective and timely way, we need to take account of some of the problems for patients and staff at this transition point.

Above all the techniques and approaches we have mentioned, we have the best chance of helping our patients and their families by: trying to understand what *they* think, and working closely and relying on our colleagues from different professions and different teams. The transition to palliative care is much more than a referral process between differing disciplines.[19] It involves the patient and family in readjusting their hopes and expectations and working in partnership with healthcare professionals.

References

1 Ashby, M. and Stofell, B. (1991). Therapeutic ratio and defined phases; proposal of an ethical framework for palliative care. *BMJ* **302**, 1322–1344.

2 Jeffrey, D. (1995). Appropriate palliative care: when does it begin? *Eu J Cancer Care* **4**, 122–126.

3 Faithfull, S. (1994). The concept of cure in cancer care. *Eu J Cancer Care* **3**, 12–17.

4 World Health Organization (1990). *Cancer pain relief and palliative care: Report of a WHO Expert Committee.* Geneva.

5 National Council for Hospice and Specialist Palliative Care Services (2002). *Definitions of supportive and palliative care.* A Consultation Paper. January.

6 George, R. J. D. and Jennings, A. L. (1993). Palliative care. *Postgrad Med J* 429–449.

7 Balmer, C. E., Thomas, P., and Osborne, R. J. (2001). Who wants second-line, palliative chemotherapy? *Psycho-Oncology* **10**, 410–418.

8 Calman, K. (1988). Ethical implications of terminal care. In *Medicine, ethics and law* (ed., Freeman, M.). London.

9 Kaye, P. (1996). *Breaking bad news: a ten step approach.* EPL Publications, Northampton.

10 Jeffrey, D. (2000). *Cancer from cure to care.* Hochland and Hochland, Manchester.

11 Howie, J. G. R. *et al.* (1999). Quality at general practice consultations: crossectional survey. *BMJ* **319**, 738–43.

12 British Medical Association (BMA) (2002). *Withholding and withdrawing life-prolonging medical treatment. Guidance for decision making* (2nd edn). BMA, London.

13 Reid, C. and Jeffrey, D. (2002). Do not attempt resuscitation decisions in a cancer centre: addressing difficult ethical and communication issues. *Br J Cancer* **86**, 1057–1060.

14 British Medical Association (BMA), The Resuscitation Council (UK) and The Royal College of Nursing (2001). *Decisions relating to cardiopulmonary resuscitation: a joint statement.*

15 Leventhal, H., Meyer, D., and Nevenz, D. (1980). The commonsense representation of illness danger, in *Medical Psychology 2* (ed., S. Rackman) pp. 7–30. New York, Pergamon.

16 Ajzen, I. (1985). From intentions to actions: a theory of planned behaviour. In *Action control: from cognition to behavior* (ed., Kuhl, J. and Beckman, J.) pp. 11–39. Springer-Verlag, Berlin.

17 Calman, K. (1984). quality of life in cancer patients—an hypothesis. *J Med Ethics* **10**, 124–127.

18 Kubler-Ross, E. (1970). *On Death and Dying,* London, Taristock Publications.

19 Ronaldson, S. and Devery, K. (2001). The experience of transition of palliative care services: perspectives of patients and nurses. *Int J Pall Nursing* **7**, 171–177.

Chapter 11

The significance and management of anaemia in palliative care patients

Wale Atoyebi, Tim Littlewood, and Robert Twycross

Introduction

Anaemia is a common complication of cancer and cancer therapies. This chapter will review the background, causes, investigation, and management of anaemia in the palliative care setting. The evidence-base for the approach to managing anaemia in this setting is mostly by extrapolation from studies published in the last ten years in cancer patients still receiving oncological treatment when treated for anaemia with either blood transfusion[1-3] or recombinant erythropoietin (rHuEpo).[4,5]

Scope of the problem

Anaemia in adults is defined as a haemoglobin concentration of less than 13 g/dl in men and 12 g/dl in women. It occurs in up to 50% of patients with solid tumours and in most patients with lympho-proliferative disorders, such as myeloma and lymphoma. Anaemia can give rise to various symptoms including fatigue, weakness, and dyspnoea on exertion. Such symptoms are non-specific and have not been fully investigated in relation to anaemia in terminally ill cancer patients. This is probably because they are considered integral to the general debility of end-stage disease.

Clinical assessment

Specific criteria for the clinical assessment of anaemia are lacking.[2] One of the cardinal symptoms of anaemia is fatigue. It is defined as a general feeling of debilitating tiredness or loss of energy. It is a highly prevalent symptom among cancer patients and is associated with significant functional morbidity, distress and reduced quality of life (QOL).[5] The negative effect of fatigue on QOL is comparable to pain and, in some patients, it is the most debilitating symptom. Other symptoms of anaemia include impaired concentration, weakness, dyspnoea on exertion, chest pain, tachycardia, low mood, and loss of libido.[4] Randomized controlled trials of the management of cancer-related anaemia have used validated instruments in assessing the effect of anaemia on QOL. These include:

1. Linear analogue scale assessment (LASA). Also known as cancer linear analogue scale (CLAS). Consists of three linear analogue scales, each 100 mm long, and measures level of energy, the ability to do daily activities, and overall quality of life related to cancer symptoms. Patients score their own perceptions of these domains by placing a mark along the line with 0 as worst and 100 as best QOL.[6]

2. Functional assessment of cancer therapy—anaemia (FACT-An). This is a 55-item questionnaire consisting of a 34-item general questionnaire, the FACT-G and a 21-item anaemia sub-scale. Of the 21 anaemia items, 13 comprise a separate fatigue sub-scale.[7]

The LASA and FACT scales are cancer-specific and have demonstrated sensitivity to haemoglobin concentrations in large groups of patients.[4] Many studies have reported that cancer-related fatigue is frequently not mentioned by patients and not assessed routinely by physicians.[8] Consequently, it is not incorporated into the treatment plan.

Case history 11.1

AA was a 60-year-old man with myeloma diagnosed one year earlier. At an out-patient consultation he reported that he was feeling very well and commented that 'I am feeling better than at any time in the last year'. At this time AA was receiving weekly chemotherapy with cyclophosphamide and his haemoglobin concentration was 9.6 g/dl. Three days after this consultation he agreed to enter a randomized trial comparing rHuEpo with placebo. At study entry, he completed the LASA (Fig. 11.1). Most normal people score between 70 and 90 mm, and a score of under 50 mm equates to serious impairment of health. AA, who said he felt well, scored himself at around 30 mm. When questioned about the discrepancy between his symptoms and his LASA score, he reported that he did feel well compared to the previous year, but that he still had severe restrictions to his lifestyle caused by fatigue and lethargy, and this was reflected in his score.

Case history 11.1 *(continued)*

Two months later, by which time his haemoglobin concentration was 13.5 g/dl, his score on the LASA had approximately doubled to 60 mm (Fig. 11.2). This anecdote illustrates two main points. First, patients may not always freely admit all their symptoms to their doctor and it may be important to ask more specific questions. Second, correcting anaemia improved the patient's quality of life but did not return it to normal. He still had myeloma and was continuing to receive chemotherapy, both of which are likely to adversely impact on a patient's quality of life.

Differential diagnosis

Causes of anaemia in advanced malignant disease include:

- anaemia of chronic disease related to malignancy;
- concomitant chemotherapy and or radiotherapy;
- bone marrow failure;
- iron-deficiency;
- malnutrition;
- haemolytic anaemia;
- renal failure;
- chronic inflammatory disorders.

1. How would you rate your energy level during the past week?

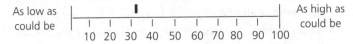

2. How would you rate your ability to do daily activities during the past week?

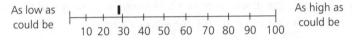

3. How would you rate your overall QOL during the past week?

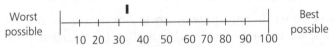

Fig. 11.1 Quality of Life (QOL)—patient assessment, pre-entry.

1. How would you rate your energy level during the past week?

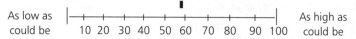

As low as could be   10 20 30 40 50 60 70 80 90 100   As high as could be

2. How would you rate your ability to do daily activities during the past week?

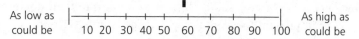

As low as could be   10 20 30 40 50 60 70 80 90 100   As high as could be

3. How would you rate your overall QOL during the past week?

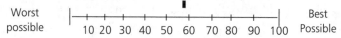

Worst possible   10 20 30 40 50 60 70 80 90 100   Best Possible

Fig. 11.2 Quality of Life (QOL)—patient assessment, week eight.

Anaemia of chronic disease in malignancy

Anaemia of chronic disease (ACD) is caused by the release of several cytokines as a reaction to malignancy or inflammation. Interleukin 1 (IL-1), tumour necrosis factor alpha (TNF-α) and γ-interferon initiate an immune response which:

◆ suppresses production and response to erythropoetin

◆ impairs transferrin production, resulting in reduced availability of stored iron

◆ shortens red cell survival.

Bone marrow failure

Bone marrow failure may be caused by extensive treatment with myelotoxic chemotherapy and/or radiotherapy or, sometimes, the presence of tumour or fibrosis involving the bone marrow. Pancytopenia and a leucoerythroblastic peripheral smear is suggestive of metastatic disease within the marrow. The need to make a firm diagnosis of marrow infiltration by tumour has to be balanced against the discomfort of a bone marrow biopsy and the lack of therapeutic options for metastatic bone marrow disease.

Iron-deficiency anaemia

Acute and chronic haemorrhage occurs in 20% of patients with advanced cancer, and is a major cause of morbidity. Bleeding contributes to death in 5% of patients.

Malnutrition

As a result of a poor diet, which is common in severely ill patients with cancer, dietary deficiency of haematologically important nutrients, such as vitamin B_{12} and folic acid, can occur. Folate antagonists, such as methotrexate, can also cause folate deficiency. Folate deficiency will present as a macrocytic anaemia. Chronic protein malnutrition can lead to generalised hypoproteinaemia and marrow failure.

Haemolysis

This occurs most commonly in lymphoproliferative disorders and is usually autoimmune in origin. A micro-angiopathic haemolytic anaemia may occur in association with some forms of adenocarcinoma.

Renal failure, chronic inflammatory disorders

Many patients with cancer will have other important illnesses, which may result in anaemia. It is important to take note of these in the differential diagnosis of anaemia.

Laboratory evaluation

It is important to differentiate between iron-deficiency anaemia and anaemia of chronic disease (Table 11.1). However, these conditions may co-exist and, in any case, the anaemia may well be multifactorial in origin. Laboratory investigations need to be individualized depending on the patient's prognosis and the likelihood of remediable causes of the anaemia (Table 11.2).

Why treat anaemia in the palliative care setting?

The impact of anaemia on QOL can be considerable in cancer patients. A Canadian survey of over 900 patients, who had received cancer treatment

Table 11.1 Iron-deficiency anaemia compared with anaemia of chronic disease

	Iron-deficiency anaemia	Anaemia of chronic disease
Blood film	Hypochromic microcytic	Normochromic or hypochromic Rarely microcytic
TIBC	High	Low
Plasma iron	Low	Low
Serum ferritin	Low	Normal/high
Transferrin receptor	High	Normal

TIBC = total iron-binding capacity.

Table 11.2 Diagnostic tests in other forms of anaemia

Anaemia	Diagnosis
Bone marrow failure	Pancytopenia, bone marrow examination
Malnutrition	Serum B_{12}, red cell folate
Haemolysis	Coombs test, reticulocyte count, bilirubin, LDH
	Red cell fragmentation indicates micro-angiopathy

LDH = lactate dehydrogenase.

within the previous two years, indicated that fatigue (78%) and anxiety (77%) had been their most common symptoms, and that fatigue was the most debilitating.[9]

Approach to management

Treat iatrogenic causes

1. Discontinuation of drugs that increase bleeding risk, e.g. non-steroidal anti-inflammatory drugs and anticoagulants, and possibly corticosteroids.
2. Prescribe gastro-protective therapy, e.g. H_2-receptor antagonists and proton pump inhibitors.

Replacement of haematinic deficiencies

1. Iron-deficiency:
   (a) ferrous sulphate 200 mg b.d. or t.d.s. orally; elemental iron per tablet = 60 mg
   (b) recommended replacement therapy = 100–200 mg elemental iron/day
   (c) alternative preparations include ferrous fumarate and ferrous gluconate.
2. Folate deficiency: folic acid 5 mg o.d..
3. Vitamin B_{12} deficiency: hydroxycobalamin 1000 μg every 3 months intramuscularly.

Vitamin K replacement therapy in liver disease and malabsorption

Vitamin K 5–10 mg subcutaneously with prothrombin time monitoring.

Tranexamic acid as an antifibrinolytic agent in mucosal bleeding

Tranexamic acid 10 mg/kg intravenously every 4 h or 15 mg/kg orally every 8 h.

Blood transfusion

Blood transfusion as a supportive treatment in haematology and oncology is well established. Few studies have looked at its benefit in terminally ill patients.

A retrospective audit looked at over 100 patients who received 143 transfusions over a 7-year period in a palliative care unit.[10] Weakness was reported by 81%, dyspnoea by 54%, and fatigue by 24%. Within one week 9% died, and 34% within four weeks of transfusion. During the patient's terminal admission, 30/143 (21%) transfusions were given.

A multicentre prospective audit evaluated the subjective benefits of transfusion in over 90 palliative care patients.[3] Common causes of anaemia were anaemia of chronic disease (54%), chronic haemorrhage (21%), and marrow infiltration (21%), although the criteria for confirming the cause were unspecified. All the patients reported weakness and 41% complained of dyspnoea. Nearly one-third of the patients died within 2 weeks of transfusion. In those who survived, there was a statistically significant improvement in strength, dyspnoea, and well-being after transfusion. However, the pre-transfusion haemoglobin concentration did not predict symptoms of anaemia or response to transfusion.

Another palliative care unit reported on the experience of blood transfusion in some 250 consecutive terminally ill inpatients; one or more blood transfusions were given to 12% of the patients.[3] Half reported improvement in well-being after transfusion. Once again pre-transfusion haemoglobin concentration and the severity of pre-transfusion symptoms were not predictive of the response to transfusion. Non-responders had a statistically significant reduction in survival, and 60% of the transfusion recipients died during the same admission.

When to transfuse?

Terminally ill cancer patients are reported to be at high risk of inappropriate transfusions because the decision to transfuse is often based on a single haemoglobin measurement.[11] However, the most important factor in determining the need for a transfusion in a chronically anaemic patient is the presence or absence of symptoms attributable to the anaemia. In the presence of symptoms such as dyspnoea, angina, postural hypotension, headache, or pulmonary oedema with no alternative explanation, a trial transfusion is indicated. Patients with chronic anaemia of slow onset tolerate levels of haemoglobin much lower than those tolerated by patients after acute haemorrhage. The progression of anaemia in the palliative care setting can also be anticipated. In cancer patients with anaemia, transfusions are usually prescribed when the haemoglobin is below 8–9 g/dl. One unit of packed red cells results in the haemoglobin rise of 1 g/dl, therefore a 3–4 unit transfusion will raise the haemoglobin concentration to 11–12 g/dl. Each unit provides 270 ± 50 ml of fluid; three units therefore potentially provides in excess of 900 ml of fluid. This volume cannot be tolerated over a short period by some patients. The administration of a small amount of diuretic (furosemide 20 mg with alternate units) might be required. Each unit is administered over 2–4 h.

When not to transfuse?

The following are all contra-indications to further blood transfusion:

- if a patient prefers not to be transfused
- no benefit from previous transfusion
- patient is moribund with a life-expectancy of days
- if the transfusion can best be described as simply prolonging a patient's death.

Some of the uncertainties relating to the question of transfusion are illustrated in Case history 11.2.[12]

Case history 11.2

MM, a 62-year-old woman, was diagnosed as having lymphoma within a year of treatment for cancer of the colon. Although chemotherapy was initially successful, the lymphoma recurred and further aggressive treatment was deemed inappropriate. After the change to palliative care, she began to plan a party, which she said would be 'more important than my funeral'. This took place two months later, bringing together her family, friends, and neighbours. She required several transfusions for recurrent gastro-intestinal bleeding to keep her going. More blood two days before the party gave her the boost she needed. Then her relatives dispersed, leaving a sister to care for her. Most of her affairs were in order. She completed her funeral arrangements and began to live in one room in her home, in a limbo of waiting.

Case history 11.2 *(continued)*

'Nothing went right from then on', she said later. She again became weak and breathless from anaemia, and was repeatedly transfused. An abdominal mass enlarged and she had episodes of intestinal obstruction. She grew impatient with the 'nil by mouth and drip' regimen. She tried to tell her consultant that death from anaemia would be preferable to the state she was in and that she saw no point in transfusions now that the benefit was so brief. Her sister reluctantly returned home. Then MM had melaena and, despite being almost moribund, was given five units of blood. She stayed in hospital awaiting a vacancy in the palliative care unit. Ten days later she was transferred and died within hours, two months after the party.

With her family's encouragement, a retired psycho-oncologist arranged to see her consultant, in the hope that lessons might be learned from MM's suffering. Together they identified that there were two main issues: communication and the use of blood transfusions. Reasons for the breakdown in communication included her loyalty and gratitude, which inhibited her criticism; failure to monitor her wishes as the illness progressed; and failure to include social factors in making clinical decisions. The consultant remarked, 'It seems she was crying out to die and we missed it'.

On the question of blood transfusion, they could not reach agreement. Although he would have been willing to withhold antibiotics at her request, he was unwilling to let anyone die of acute blood loss. He mentioned that the ethical issues involved in letting someone die in this way could be stressful and divisive for his team. He explained that failure to treat acute anaemia could be unpleasant for the patient, causing air hunger and dehydration, and that it carried a risk of cortical blindness. In contrast, a palliative care specialist subsequently consulted informally, thought that MM could have been kept comfortable relatively easily without the use of blood, and could have died peacefully.

Response to transfusion

Of patients who have been transfused, 50–75% obtain some benefit in terms of well-being, strength, and breathlessness.[2,3,11]

Limitations of blood transfusions

Blood transfusions do not always achieve benefit, and sometimes harm the patient. Limitations include:

◆ inconvenient and time-consuming

◆ transient benefit

◆ volume overload

◆ allergic reaction risk

◆ haemolytic reactions

◆ infection risk

◆ limited supply of blood.

Recombinant erythropoietin

The use of rHuEPO is an alternative option to blood transfusion for anaemic patients with cancer, and was first reported in patients with advanced multiple myeloma.[13] There have been no randomized studies looking at the use of rHuEPO specifically in palliative care.

Mechanism of action of rHuEPO

Erythropoietin is a glycoprotein hormone that is a primary regulator of erythropoiesis, maintaining the body's red cell mass at an optimal level. In response to a decrease in tissue oxygenation, erythropoietin synthesis increases in the kidney. The secreted hormone binds to specific receptors on the surface of the red cell precursors in the bone marrow, leading to their survival, proliferation, and differentiation, and ultimately to an increase in haematocrit. Since its introduction more than a decade ago, rHuEPO has become the standard of care in treating the anaemia associated with chronic renal failure. It has also been approved for the treatment of anaemia associated with cancer and HIV infection, and for use in the surgical setting to reduce the need for allogeneic blood transfusions. For all indications it is well tolerated and efficacious.

Available erythropoietin preparations

◆ Epoetin alfa

◆ epoetin beta

◆ darbepoetin alpha (novel erythropoiesis stimulating protein).

These three recombinant erythropoietin preparations differ in terms of sialic acid containing carbohydrate content within the molecule. Darbepoetin alfa has an increased serum half-life and *in vivo* biological activity compared to epoetin alfa and beta.

Guidelines for epoetin administration

Epoetin (alfa and beta) 150–300 iu/kg subcutaneously three times a week leads to:

- an increase in haemoglobin of 2 g/dl or increase in haematocrit of >6% in 50–60% of patients
- improved QOL with each increment in haemoglobin up to a level of around 11–12 g/dl
- reduction in transfusion need by approximately 50%, excluding transfusions required during the first month of treatment before rHuEPO has had time to work.

Recent prospective studies of a once-weekly dosing regimen (40 000–60 000 units) of epoetin alfa in patients, has shown improvements in haemoglobin and QOL similar to three-times weekly dosing.[14] Darbepoetin alpha is currently undergoing clinical trials in the setting of cancer-related anaemia; it is administered once weekly at a dose of 4.5 μg/kg.

Undesirable effects of rHuEPO include:

- hypertension
- polycythaemia
- anti-erythropoetin antibodies.

An excessive increase in red cell mass is avoided by reducing the dose by 25% if the haemoglobin concentration rises by >2 g/dl per month, and by aiming to maintain a haemoglobin of 11 g/dl in women and 12 g/dl in men. A recent report has described the development of anti-erythropoetin antibodies in patients with renal failure treated with rHuEPO. All the patients affected developed red cell aplasia. The cause is unclear but may be related to differences in the carbohydrate content of recombinant and naturally occurring erythropoetin. If antibodies are detected, treatment with erythropoetin must be discontinued; switching to an alternative formulation is contra-indicated.

Limitations of rHuEPO

1. Effective in only 50–60% of patients.
2. Inconvenience of rHuEPO. This may be of great importance to patients. A three-times weekly schedule may be difficult from a compliance perspective, but the benefit of home administration and the longer-acting preparations might overcome this to a certain extent.
3. Response can take four weeks or longer. This could lead to termination of therapy with rHuEPO prematurely due to a lack of perceived benefit.
4. No adequate predictors of response. Although numerous variables (haemoglobin, serum erythropoietin levels, ferritin, CRP, transferrin,

Table 11.3 Comparison of blood transfusion and erythropoietin

	rHuEPO	Transfusion
Inconvenience to patient	SC injection	IV infusion
Speed of effect	4–6 weeks	Immediate
Rise in haemoglobin	Prolonged	Transient
Safety	Adverse effects rare and generally minor	Risk of transfusion reactions and infections

transferrin receptor, serum iron, haematocrit, and reticulocytes) measured after 2 weeks have been found to significantly correlate with response, none is associated strongly enough to serve as a reliable single prognostic indicator. If serum erythropoietin concentration is less than 100 mU/ml and haemoglobin concentration is increased by >0.5 g/dl after 2 weeks of treatment, the patient is very likely to respond to the current dose (predictive power 95%).

5. Concurrent iron-deficiency. A common cause of limited response to erythropoietin.

Several issues still need to be addressed before firm recommendations on the use of rHuEPO in the palliative care setting can be made (Table 11.3). These include optimal dose and schedule, when to increase the dose, and when to stop the drug because of lack of response.

Relative cost: blood transfusions versus rHuEPO

Red cell transfusions have historically been viewed as less expensive than rHuEPO. However, it is difficult to gain a current accurate measurement of the cost of acquiring, handling, processing, storing, and administering blood. There are also the costs associated with the complications of transfusions and the indirect economic costs to patients due to travelling to have blood transfused.

Unresolved issues

Identifying, monitoring, and effectively treating anaemic patients in the palliative care setting is not an easy task. Studies in patients treated with rHuEPO have demonstrated a non-linear relationship between haemoglobin concentration and QOL.[15] The largest QOL improvement occurred when the haemoglobin increased above 11–12 g/dl, whereas little benefit was noted when the haemoglobin increased between 7 and 8 g/dl. Thus, a haemoglobin concentration below 11 g/dl may be an appropriate trigger point for intervention in those patients whose symptoms have not already necessitated intervention. However both symptoms and haemoglobin concentration should be considered when making treatment decisions, but the relative value to be placed on each item remains to be defined. Ideally, patients should not have to wait until their anaemia becomes debilitating before receiving treatment.

References

1 Barrett-Lee, P. J., Bailey, N. P., O'Brien, M. E. *et al.* (2000). Large-scale UK audit of blood transfusion requirements and anaemia in patients receiving cytotoxic chemotherapy. *Br J Cancer* **82**, 93–97.

2 Monti, M., Castellani, L., Berlusconi, A. *et al.* (1996). Use of red blood cell transfusions in terminally ill cancer patients admitted to a palliative care unit. *J Pain Symptom Manage* **12**, 8–22.

3 Gleeson, C. and Spencer, D. (1995). Blood transfusion and its benefits in palliative care. *Palliat Med* **9**, 307–313.

4 Littlewood, T. J., Bajetta, E., Nortier, J. W. *et al.* (2001). Effects of epoetin alfa on hematologic parameters and quality of life in cancer patients receiving nonplatinum chemotherapy: results of a randomized, double-blind, placebo-controlled trial. *J Clin Oncol* **19**, 2865–2874.

5 Quirt, I., Robeson, C., Lau, C. Y. *et al.* (2001). Epoetin alfa therapy increases hemoglobin levels and improves quality of life in patients with cancer-related anemia who are not receiving chemotherapy and patients with anemia who are receiving chemotherapy. *J Clin Oncol* **19**, 4126–4134.

6 Holmes, S. and Dickerson, J. (1987). The quality of life: design and evaluation of a self-assessment instrument for use with cancer patients. *Int J Nurs Stud* **24**, 15–24.

7 Cella, D. (1997). The Functional Assessment of Cancer Therapy-Anaemia (FACT-An) scale: a new tool for the assessment of outcomes in cancer anemia and fatigue. *Semin Hematol* **34**, 13–19 (suppl 2).

8 Turner, A. R. (1998). Symptom Management. In *Oxford textbook of palliative care* (2nd edn) (ed., Doyle, D., Hanks, G. W. C., and MacDonald, N.), pp. 769–772. Oxford University Press, Oxford.

9 Ashbury, F. D., Findlay, H., Reynolds, B. *et al.* (1998). A Canadian survey of cancer patients' experiences: are their needs being met? *J Pain Symptom Manage* **16**, 298–306.

10 Chambers, J. (2002). *Do our prescribing habits influence the need for blood transfusions in the Hospice.* Abstract of poster presented at palliative care congress, Sheffield, UK.

11 Sciortino, A. D., Carlton, D. C., Axelrod, A. *et al.* (1993). The efficacy of administering blood transfusions at home to terminally ill cancer patients. *J Palliat Care* **9**, 14–17.

12 Stedeford, A. (2001). An indestructible patient. *BMJ* **57**, 323.

13 Ludwig, H., Fritz, E., Kotzmann, H. *et al.* (1990). Erythropoietin treatment of anemia associated with multiple myeloma. *N Engl J Med* **322**, 1693–1699.

14 Gabrilove, J. L., Cleeland, C. S., Livingston, R. B. *et al.* (2001). Clinical evaluation of once-weekly dosing of epoetin alfa in chemotherapy patients: improvements in hemoglobin and quality of life are similar to three-times-weekly dosing. *J Clin Oncol* **19**, 2875–2882.

15 Cleeland, C. S., Demetri, G. D., Glaspy, J. *et al.* (1999). Identifying haemoglobin level for optimal quality of life: results of an incremental analysis. *Proc Am Soc Clin Oncol* **18**, 2215a.

Chapter 12

Thrombotic and bleeding complications in haematological malignancies

Beverley Hunt and Simon Noble

Introduction

Venous thrombo-embolism and bleeding problems are common complications of advanced malignancy and have been recognized since the original descriptions of migratory thrombophlebitis associated with adenocarcinoma by Trousseau more than 100 years ago. This chapter will concentrate on the management of thrombotic and bleeding complications in patients with haematological malignancies, for whom further curative treatment is no longer possible or appropriate.

The pathogenesis of some disorders such as thrombocytopenia, following marrow infiltration, is easily understood. However, other haemostatic effects may be more directly related to the malignant process as outlined in Table 12.1.

The transition from active treatment to comfort-only is sometimes a difficult one to make. Many times before, the team may have witnessed the same patient brought back from near death by treating situations such as severe sepsis and disseminated intravascular coagulation (DIC). Such intense

Table 12.1 Tumour-related haemostatic effects in haematology

- Release of thromboplastic substances causing DIC or vascular thrombosis, e.g. acute promyelocytic leukaemia.
- Megakaryocytic involvement in malignant transformation leading to dysfunctional platelets, e.g. chronic myeloproliferative disorders.
- Abnormal lymphocytes or plasma cells producing proteins that interfere with haemostasis, e.g. multiple myeloma.
- Drug-induced thrombosis or bleeding, e.g. L-asparginase or B-lactam antibiotics.

management at the end-stage of life, when futile, may obstruct the provision of patient dignity and comfort. The needs of the family in bereavement will also be affected by how they perceived, and perhaps witnessed, their loved one's death. A family may, in years to come, perceive being ushered from the room, as the team 'did all they could' for their loved one, with resentment and regret, feeling that they were denied the opportunity to be with them when they died. However, the changing role of the palliative-care team, in particular as part of the support team within an acute hospital, means that more often we are considering palliative-care patients for aggressive supportive treatments.

The importance of identifying patients for whom comfort measures, and no further active treatment, are appropriate cannot be over emphasized. Team planning can identify and anticipate complications that may arise and establish plans for each one. These will need to be individualized for each patient depending upon their clinical situation, vascular access, and so on. Hickman line and patient ambitions, e.g. desire to be at home, previous objective and symptomatic response to a therapy, e.g. platelet transfusion, may guide the team in further planning.

This chapter will concentrate more on the symptomatic control of thrombotic and haemorrhagic complications. In practice, within the field of palliative care, the management of these complications is dealt with separately, since symptom control at the end of life tends to focus on the most distressing symptoms first. Often the treatment options may not be appropriate to the patient's current clinical state and teams will need to be flexible in adapting treatment plans for each patient.

Venous thrombo-embolism

Cancer is a major risk factor for venous thrombo-embolism (VTE): it is estimated that almost 15% of cancer patients will have a thrombo-embolic event. Cancer patients have a high risk of VTE after surgery and chemotherapy may potentiate the risk. Haematological cancers are amongst the most prothrombotic of malignancies and population studies have demonstrated them to have a greater risk than colon, lung, and breast cancers.[1] One study has shown that of all the oncology patients, palliative care in-patients have an even higher risk of VTE, with a deep vein thrombosis (DVT) prevalence as high as 52%. Of these, 33% were found to have bilateral DVTs.[2] Clinically they may be asymptomatic, but they often result in painful swollen legs. The more extreme cases result in severe disability and vascular insufficiency. Pulmonary embolism (PE) is a well-recognized complication but is often not pursued diagnostically in the palliative-care setting because of difficulties in accurate imaging and access to facilities. Sometimes an active decision is made 'not to treat'. Nevertheless, 30% of those with proven DVT later develop symptoms suggestive of PE and many sudden unexpected deaths in specialist palliative-care units (SPCUs) are assumed to be related to thrombo-embolism.[2] It has recently been recognized that some forms of chemotherapy are associated with increased risk of VTE. The most recently described is thalidomide, which is being used increasingly to treat immunosecretory disorders.

Prothrombotic changes associated with haematological malignancies

Virchow's triad describes the predisposing factors for VTE, namely: stasis, changes in the vessel wall, and changes in the blood. Table 12.2 summarizes the features that predispose oncology patients to a high risk of thrombosis. There are specific abnormalities associated with cancer patients:

1. Tumour procoagulants have been identified and are complied on the International Society for Thrombosis and Haemostasis registry. The two principal tumour cell procoagulants are: tissue factor and cancer procoagulant. The latter directly activates factor X in the absence of factor VII. The tumour cell procoagulants are probably responsible for cases of Trousseau's syndrome. In 1865 Trousseau first described the association of migratory thrombophlebitis and gastric carcinoma. Unlike the more common, solitary, deep vein thromboses that affect the legs, the phlebitis of Trousseau's syndrome is recurrent and migratory, and it affects both the superficial and

Table 12.2 Risk factors for thrombosis

◆ **Stasis**:
—immobility
—extrinsic pressure, e.g. oedematous limbs.

◆ **Vessel wall/endothelial perturbation**:
—cytokine release from tumours
—local tumour infiltration
—central venous catheter.

◆ **Hypercoagualability**:
—dehydration
—cytokine-related prothrombotic changes
—tissue factor/cancer procoagulant expression on tumour
  cells
—DIC
—increased platelet activation.

deep vein systems. Unusual sites such as arms, neck, as well as superficial veins of the thorax and abdomen may be involved. Typically such a patient has an occult tumour, usually adenocarcinoma; although up to 10% may have an acute leukaemia. It is notoriously difficult to treat. In the authors' experience the combination of high dose warfarin with full-dose LMW heparin +/− aspirin may still not control the thrombotic tendency.

2. Antiphospholipid antibodies. These acquired antibodies are associated with thrombosis. They are detected by performing a lupus anticoagulant assay and anticardiolipin antibody, both of which must be performed, as only one may be positive. The antibody must be demonstrated on two separate occasions more than 6 weeks apart. The antiphospholipid syndrome is the association of the antibody with thrombosis or pregnancy morbidity.

Thrombotic complications can occur in any vessel be it arterial, venous or microvascular. If these patients have a significant thrombosis they should receive standard heparin and then high-dose warfarin therapy (INR 3–4). The syndrome has been reported in association with myeloma and related disorders. The antiphospholipid antibody (it is said) may disappear with successful treatment of the underlying disorder, although this is not the authors' personal experience.

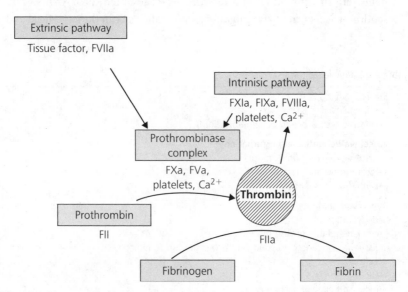

Fig. 12.1 The coagulation cascade.

Management of venous thrombo-embolism

The aims of treatment of thrombo-embolism in the palliative care setting are as follows:

- decrease symptoms, e.g. pain, swelling, dyspnoea
- prevent thrombus propagation
- prevent imminent death
- minimize untoward side-effects of treatment.

Treatment plans need to be individualized for each patient and risk/benefit ratios assessed. Of active treatment options available, providing the patient has a reasonably normal coagulation screen and a platelet count greater than $75 \times 10^9/l$ (an unusual finding in those with haematological malignancies), then conventional management with compression stockings and treatment doses of low molecular weight heparin (LMWH) is most likely to achieve symptom control and prevent further thrombotic events. If the patient stabilizes, then conversion to oral anticoagulation can be considered. Each of these drugs has their own burden of risks that need to be considered in advanced haematological malignancy. The majority of patients, however, are significantly thrombocytopenic and thus the dose of LMW heparin has to be modified. If the patient's platelet count is $<20 \times 10^9/l$, it is contra-indicated due to the associated risks of bleeding, and management has to be limited to conservative measures such as using anti-thrombo-embolic stockings.

Low molecular weight heparin

LMWHs are being evaluated as an alternative to oral anticoagulants for long-term therapy in cancer patients. Their mechanism of action is shown in Fig. 12.2. They are thought to be more advantageous for several reasons:[3]

- LMWH have reliable pharmacokinetics and thus unlike unfractionated heparin, do not require laboratory monitoring
- a more uniform anticoagulant response is achieved because, unlike current oral anticoagulants, diet and concomitant drugs do not influence their anticoagulant effect
- rapid onset of action.

To date, several randomized studies have compared oral anticoagulant therapy with LMWH for long-term treatment of VTE. In these studies, the incidence of bleeding was similar in the two treatment groups. However, it should be noted that cancer patients (and even fewer haemato-oncology patients) accounted for only a small proportion of the study samples.[4]

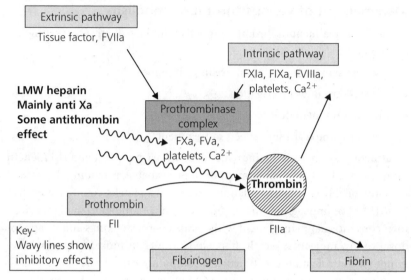

Fig. 12.2 Site of action of low molecular weight heparin (LMWH).

Oral anticoagulation

Although warfarin is the mainstay of long-term anticoagulation for VTE, several studies have demonstrated significant increases in rates of bleeding amongst cancer patients receiving oral anticoagulation (as high as 21.6% in one study).[5] Their inhibitory effects on coagulation are shown in Fig. 12.3. Within the palliative-care setting, in patients with far more advanced disease, the bleeding incidence was higher, even with strict monitoring of anticoagulation.[6] Factors such as thrombocytopenia and liver disease will further increase the risk of bleeding. The decision to use warfarin or one of its analogues should not be undertaken lightly in patients with haematological malignancies, for safe anticoagulation will require intensive monitoring of the INR and the burden of repeated blood tests.

Future oral anticoagulation

A new type of oral anticoagulant is currently in phase III studies and should be licensed initially for thromboprophylaxis in orthopaedic surgery in 2003. These oral direct-thrombin inhibitors potentially offer the prospect of a new age in anticoagulation: oral anticoagulation that is efficacious and that will not require monitoring due to their predictable pharmacokinetics. These drugs therefore hold great promise in the management of VTE in cancer patients.

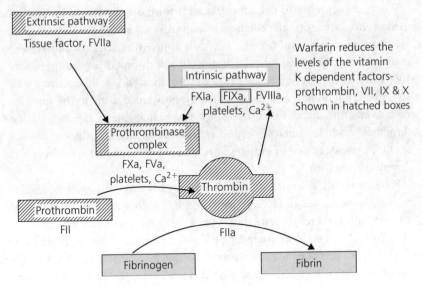

Fig. 12.3 Site of action of warfarin.

Vena caval filters

These are appropriate when recurrent pulmonary emboli occur despite effective anticoagulation, or where anticoagulation is not possible. They are rarely used in the palliative-care patient group but may be considered in exceptional circumstances.[7]

Thromboprophylaxis

It is the authors' contention that due to the high risk of VTE in palliative-care patients, and the severe symptoms that can result from VTE, there is a strong argument for using thromboprophylaxis in this group, although there are few studies in this area. Several LMW heparins are licensed for thromboprophylaxis in 'medical' patients, which one could argue covers the area of palliative care.

Catheter-related thrombosis

Long-term indwelling central venous catheters (CVCs) are commonly used for the administration of chemotherapy, parenteral nutrition, and blood products and for drawing blood. Up to 60% of patients with CVCs will develop a complication secondary to the device, thrombosis being one of the most common. Thrombosis associated with a CVC may involve the catheter tip, the length of the catheter, the catheterized vessel in the upper limb, the central vasculature of the neck/mediastinum, or a combination of these.

The true incidence of catheter-related thrombosis is uncertain. Studies using venography for surveillance or diagnosis suggested the incidence of asymptomatic and symptomatic events is approximately 40% and 10% of patients with CVCs, respectively, or one clinical thrombotic event per every 1000 catheter days. A higher incidence of thrombosis is seen in catheters with larger external lumens and those with a tip positioned distal to the superior vena cava. Other factors that predispose to a higher rate of catheter-related thrombosis include catheter infection, infusion of sclerosing chemotherapeutic agents, extrinsic vessel compression, and a previous history of venous thrombo-embolism.

Patients with CVC-related thrombosis may present with swelling and/or pain of the arm, neck, or face. Some may present with symptoms suggestive of a PE or with catheter malfunction. Many of the symptoms are non-specific and, for this reason, objective testing is needed. Contrast venography remains the reference standard for diagnosis of CVC-related thrombosis but this is invasive and may be painful. Some centres perform line-ograms by injecting contrast dye into the catheter, using fluoroscopy to follow the flow of contrast. Studies have suggested this is a less sensitive way of diagnosing CVC-related thrombus. Venous ultrasonography, whilst highly sensitive and specific for diagnosing symptomatic lower limb DVT, has not been subjected to sufficiently rigorous studies in upper limb DVT diagnosis. However the best available evidence suggests that ultrasonography is the most accurate non-invasive test with a sensitivity and specificity of 93% and 95%, respectively.

Two open-label, randomized studies have been performed to evaluate the safety and efficacy of prophylactic anticoagulation in patients with CVCs. One study randomized patients to receive low dose warfarin (1 mg) or no treatment.[8] Venography was performed at day 90 or sooner if symptoms warranted. Of the control group, 37% compared to 10% of the warfarin group had thrombosis ($P < 0.001$). There was no difference in bleeding rates although 10% of the warfarin group required reversal of prolonged INRs with vitamin K. Another randomized trial of similar design compared 2500u dalteparin s/c once daily to no treatment.[9] The study was terminated early by the safety committee because of the large difference in thrombotic rates between groups. Of 16 patients receiving LMWH, one (6%) developed thrombosis compared to eight of 13 (62%) in the control group ($P = 0.002$). Despite these trials, most clinicians do not routinely prescribe thromboprophylaxis in cancer patients with CVCs. Larger trials are ongoing but to date none are directly comparing these two forms of prophylaxis.

Treatment of CVC-related thrombosis remains a poorly studied area. There are several treatment options available: anticoagulation alone, systemic thrombolysis, low dose local thrombolysis, catheter removal, no treatment at all, or any combination of the above.

Initial anticoagulation with LMW heparin and then warfarin appears a logical management strategy. Anticoagulation is recommended for at least three months and should be continued until after the catheter is removed. Systemic thrombolysis may cause bleeding and should be avoided. If a patient has a continued need for central venous access, a functioning catheter does not have to be removed. There is no evidence to suggest that removing the CVC will accelerate thrombus resolution or reduce complications.

Bleeding complications

The causes of bleeding in cancer patients are summarised in Table 12.3. Thrombocytopenia is common in patients with haematological malignancies due to the failure of the bone marrow to produce platelets due to the presence of disease and/or the effects of cytotoxic treatment.

Causes of thrombocytopenia

1. Lack of production. The most common cause in cancer. Due either to marrow involvement in the disease and/or the use of cytotoxic chemotherapy.
2. Excessive destruction. Thrombocytopenia due to increased peripheral destruction may be associated with DIC, drug-induced haemolytic-uraemic

Table 12.3 Haemostatic factors that contribute to bleeding

Platelets

♦ Thrombocytopenia:

—lack of production—secondary to chemotherapy
  or marrow infiltration

—consumtion—DIC, autoimmune

—hypersplenism.

♦ Abnormal function as seen in:

—acute myeloid leukaemia

—myelodysplasia

—myeloproliferative disorders

—lymphoid leukaemia's (less common)

—paraproteinaemias.

Coagulation

♦ High-level expression of tissue factor or tumour procoagulant
  leading to DIC.

♦ acquired factor inhibitors

syndrome, and autoimmunity. Immune thrombocytopenia has been rarely described with solid tumours but is clearly observed in the lymphoproliferative disorders, particularly Hodgkin's disease, chronic lymphatic leukaemia, and low-grade lymphoma. A worsening thrombocytopenia in the course of a lympho-proliferative disorder may signify an immune mechanism. Diagnosis may be difficult, particularly in cases with extensive coexisting marrow involvement, and is supported by: acute onset, large platelet size, higher than anticipated megakaryocyte number, and increased platelet-associated immunoglobulin; however, the latter finding is non-specific and inconsistent. Treatment with corticosteroids or intravenous gammaglobulin is effective. Splenectomy, further immunosuppression, danazol, treatment of *H. pylori* infection and vincristine are second line therapies.

3. Splenic pooling/hypersplenism is an occasional cause of thrombocytopenia in lymphoma and chronic lymphatic leukaemia. The thrombocytopenia related to hypersplenism is usually a mild platelet count of 40 000–100 000 $\times$ 10⁹/l and rarely causes significant bleeding.

At this present time the most effective therapy for severe thrombocytopenia due to lack of production, is platelet transfusion.

Platelet transfusion

Currently, platelets are prepared by plateletpheresis from individual donors. They are much better quality than those of 20 years ago and are viable for up to 5 days due to the use of special storage bags. Platelets awaiting use in blood transfusion are stored at room temperature and gently agitated to maintain maximum function.

As a rule of thumb, an average platelet pool should produce an increment of platelet count of 50 $\times$ 10⁹/l in a 70-kg adult, although this may not occur if the individual has antiplatelet antibodies as in idiopathic thrombocytopenic purpura.

Some patients have HLA antibodies, which can also prevent a satisfactory increment after platelet transfusion and may also cause mild transfusion reactions—usually multifarious women or exposure to previous blood components. HLA antibodies are formed following exposure to allogenic leucocytes, this was more common prior to the universal practice of leucodepletion in the UK transfusion centres. Leucodepletion was introduced in the UK in response to concerns about the potential transmission of variant-CJD, but the reduced exposure to leucocytes has also reduced transfusion reactions.

Indications for platelet transfusion

1. **Management of bleeding.** Ideally in an actively bleeding patient, the platelet count should be kept above $50 \times 10^9/l$.

2. **Prophylactic transfusion.** The main use of platelet transfusion is in the prevention of bleeding in patients with haematological malignancies (particularly leukaemias) who have bone marrow failure caused by their disease or treatment. For patients with bone marrow failure, it has been accepted practice to transfuse platelets where the levels are very low. A platelet threshold of $10 \times 10^9/l$ is as safe as higher levels for treating most patients without additional risk factors. These risk factors, including sepsis, concurrent use of drugs (e.g. antibiotics), and other abnormalities of haemostasis, are indications for a higher threshold. Higher threshold numbers are also needed to cover invasive procedures, e.g. line insertions and biopsies. The avoidance of a low haematocrit in patients with thrombocytopenia or disordered platelet function reduces the risk of haemorrhage.

3. **Patients who are refractory to platelet transfusions.** Failure to achieve a satisfactory response to platelet transfusions (refractoriness) occurs in up to half of those receiving prophylactic transfusions. This is defined by the poor increment in platelet count rather than on clinical grounds. Satisfactory increments are frequently obtained by the use of HLA-matched platelets, but their effectiveness in reducing severe bleeding deserves more detailed evaluation.

Unusual bleeding problems seen in immunosecretory malignancies

Unique derangements of haemostasis occur in association with the immunosecretory and associated B-cell disorders. These are often difficult to diagnose and treat; the input of a haemostatic expert in both, is vital. They are listed in Table 12.4 and described below:

Clinical bleeding in B-cell malignancies

Various haemostatic abnormalities can be detected in patients with either multiple myeloma or Waldenstrom's macroglobulinaemia. Clinically significant bleeding has been described in approximately 15% of patients with IgG myeloma and up to 60% of Waldenstrom's macroglobulinaemia, due to the interaction of the paraprotein with clotting factors and platelets—simplistically, the paraprotein coats the clotting factors and platelets, preventing their interactions. The extent of the bleeding disease appears to correlate with the

Table 12.4 Haemostatic abnormalities in immunosecretory disorders

Haemorrhagic

Secondary to paraprotein:

- acquired von Willebrand's syndrome
- amyloidosis (factor X deficiency)
- platelet function defects due to paraprotein coating platelets
- fibrin defects due to paraprotein coating fibrin
- circulating anticoagulants.

Unrelated to paraprotein:

- thrombocytopenia due to marrow infiltration
- renal disease
- disseminated intravascular coagulation.

Thrombotic

Related to paraprotein:

- antiphospholipid antibody formation
- hyperviscosity.

Unrelated to paraprotein:

- immobility
- hypercalcaemia
- disseminated intravascular coagulation.

Table 12.5 Indications for blood products

Fresh frozen plasma

- Disseminated intravascular coagulation
- Rapid correction of warfarin overdose
- Liver disease
- Coagulopathy due to massive blood loss

Cryoprecipitate

- As a source of fibrinogen in disseminated intravascular coagulation
- For bleeding in cases of dysfibrinogenaemia

magnitude of the paraprotein level. Massive haemorrhage is the cause of death in up to 3% of myeloma patients and 9% of lymphoproliferative disorders.

The bleeding in patients with paraproteins may be in unusual sites, e.g. can cause deafness due to inner ear bleeding, periorbital ecchymoses, and intraperitoneal or retroperitoneal bleeding. Such patients are particularly prone to bleeding after invasive procedures.

The pathophysiology of such haemorrhagic disorders is often multifactoral—the aetiological factors are listed in Table 12.4.

Acquired factor VIII inhibitors

These occur rarely but can result in a serious bleeding tendency mimicking classical haemophilia with haemarthroses and postoperative bleeding. They require management by a haemophilia consultant.

Acquired von Willebrand syndrome

Von Willebrand factor (vWF) is the ligand for platelet adhesion and carrier molecule for factor VIIIC. Patients with von Willebrand syndrome present with cutaneous and mucosal bleeding, epistaxis and gastro-intestinal bleeding. Both Type I defects (reduced levels of von Willebrand factor) and Type II defects (reduced levels of high molecular weight vWF—the most functionally active form) have been associated with immunosecretory disorders. Given the heterogeneity of the pathophysiology, it is not surprising that the degree of clinical bleeding associated with acquired von Willebrand syndrome (vWS) is variable and that in some instances no bleeding tendency is apparent.

Several therapeutic approaches have been used. Obviously the most rational approach is to treat the underlying malignancy to reduce the paraprotein level. However, when the patient reaches the palliative-care stage, such treatment is often not successful. Other therapies such as the use of DDAVP (vasopressin), plasma exchange, intravenous gammaglobulin, and even extra-corporeal immunoadsorption, have been used. Replacement of vWF and Factor VIIIc with appropriate concentrate has been useful in preventing or treating bleeding. DDAVP therapy usually results in an increase in plasma vWF levels, although often due to a shortened half-life of vWF in vWS, the response may be transitory and can be expected to last for 2–4 h. In view of the tachyphalaxis seen with DDAVP, it is best reserved for the management of acute bleeding, as prophylaxis perioperatively or after a protein removal process.

Amyloid associated coagulopathies

Up to 10% of myeloma and Waldenstrom's patients develop amyloidosis. Bleeding is common with establish amyloidosis and includes petechiae, ecchymoses, gastro-intestinal bleeding, and bleeding from biopsy sites. Factor X and IX deficiency occur due to adsorption of these factors onto amyloid fibrils. This is most likely to occur in those patients whose paraprotein contains the amyloidogenic lambda VI subgroup.

The treatment of factor X and IX deficiency associated with amyloid is a challenge. Treatment of the underlying malignancy is obviously less efficacious then when compared to the approach to acquired vWD. Some success has been reported with melphalan and prednisolone. Other approaches include the use of fibrinolytic inhibitors, factor IX concentrates, and dialysis. Expert haemostatic help is required.

Abnormalities of platelet function

These are common with IgM paraproteins. Abnormalities in platelet aggregation reactions in response to various stimuli, shape change, agglutination, and release reactions have all been described; frequently more than one abnormality is present. Patients with these abnormalities present with spontaneous ecchymoses and epistaxis, or unexpected post-operative haemorrhage, despite normal coagulation studies and platelet counts. The diagnosis is confirmed with platelet function studies: either the PFA-100 (an *in vitro* assay for the bleeding time) and/or formal platelet aggregation studies.

These patients should be told to avoid aspirin and non-steroidal anti-inflammatory drugs, and other platelet modifying agents. Management of bleeding includes local compression, some patients respond to arginine vasopressin infusions. Allogenic platelet transfusion may be required in severe bleeds.

Disorders of fibrin formation

One of the first coagulation abnormalities described in B-cell disorders was impaired fibrinogen conversation to fibrin and in the polymerisation of fibrin monomers to form a stable clot. The defects are heterogeneous and result in varying degrees of haemostatic compromise.

Beyond the obvious treatment of the underlying malignancy, the use of plasmapheresis and then fibrinogen concentrates and fibrinolytic inhibitors is recommended.

Heparin-like anticoagulants

These have been described in association with dysproteinaemia, particularily plasma cell leukaemia. In these cases mucocutaneous bleeding, as well as deep haematomas, may occur. The key change is markedly prolonged thrombin time, whereas the reptilase time is normal or minimally prolonged as expected with circulating heparin-like substances. Although supportive management is the usual treatment, life-threatening continued bleeding may respond to protamine.

Vitamin K deficiency

Vitamin K deficiency as a cause of bleeding must be considered in patients with little or poor oral nutrition especially if on antibiotics.

Iatrogenic bleeding

L-asparaginase, an anti-tumour enzyme used in acute lymphoblastic leukaemia, produces marked inhibition of hepatic protein synthesis, leading to potentially pronounced depression of clotting factors synthesized by the liver. Despite prolongation of INR, PTT, and low fibrinogen levels, these patients rarely bleed and generally do not require clotting factor replacement. Occasionally thrombo-embolic complications have resulted from the low levels of antithrombin, protein C, and protein S, that are also produced by the liver.

The haemolytic uraemia syndrome—renal failure, thrombocytopenia, and a micro-angiopathic haemolytic anaemia—has been associated with cyclosporine, mitomycin-C, and occasionally cisplatin, carboplatin, and bleomycin. Pathogenesis is unclear. Early recognition with withdrawal of the drug is important for mortality from this syndrome can be up to 50%.

Myeloproliferative disorders

Bleeding and thrombosis both occur in this group of patients. Thrombosis may be in unusual sites. Bleeding has been attributed to both quantitative and qualitative platelet abnormalities, although the platelet count and bleeding time are only partially predictive of the severity and type of complication; as well as the high blood viscosity seen in polycythaemia vera.

Disseminated intravascular coagulation

Disseminated intravascular coagulation (DIC) in patients with solid tumours or leukaemia manifests as a full spectrum of clinical symptomatology. Intracranial haemorrhage, venous thrombo-embolism, and micro-angiopathic haemolysis may all be symptoms of DIC, or the patient may be asymptomatic, with laboratory abnormalities as the only manifestation of the disorder. The classic findings of thrombcytopenia, prolonged INR, and APTT, hypofib-rinogenaemia, raised levels of fibrin degradation products, and schistocytes on the blood film are uncommon. Many cancer patients have a low-grade, compensated DIC with minimally abnormal results.

Management of DIC will necessitate correction of clotting screen and platelet count by using blood products. As a simple rule of thumb, fresh frozen plasma (FFP) should be used to correct prolonged APTT and INR to ratios of <1.5; cryoprecipitate should be given if the fibrinogen level is <1 g/l, for using FFP will be unlikely to correct this. Ten bags should increase the fibrinogen level by about 1 g in a normal-sized adult. The platelet count should be kept above 50 or even 75×10^9/l by regular platelet transfusion. Antifibrinolytics should *never* be used, as they will limit the lysis of fibrin and thus the resolution of DIC. The use of heparin and antithrombin concentrates should be considered, especially if there is a low-grade or thrombotic DIC. This will limit activation and thus consumption of the clotting factors. They must be used judiciously in view of their potential to exacerbate bleeding, in conjunction with exert haemostatic help.

Complications of DIC at the end of life are more commonly haemorrhagic than thrombotic, and teams will often support patients with regular transfusions of blood products (FFP or cryoprecipitate) and platelets to prevent bleeding.

Acute promyelocytic leukaemia (APL)

This represents approximately 10–15% of acute leukaemia. The most impressive feature of APL at diagnosis is the presence in 80–90% of patients of a severe haemorrhagic syndrome, out of proportion with the degree of thrombocytopenia.[10] Mucocutaneous haemorrhages are common and before the introduction of all-trans retinoic acid (ATRA), the main cause of induction failure in APL was death from cerebral haemorrhage, with a frequency of up to 20%. The laboratory coagulation profile always shows the presence of fibrinolysis—high levels of fibrinogen/fibrin degradation products (also known as D-dimers) associated with low levels of fibrinogen and α2-antiplasm (the main plasmin inhibitor). The fibrinolytic stimulus probably relates to the abnormally high expression of annexin II on the leukaemic cells. This protein is a cell-surface receptor for plasminogen and tissue plasminogen activator. The linkage of these molecules to annexin II on the cell surface favours the activation of plasminogen to plasmin, the major fibrinolytic enzyme. The high rate of generation of plasmin results in the consumption of α2-antiplasmin, and active plasmin accumulates in the plasma favouring a haemorrhagic diathesis.

All-trans retinoic acid (ATRA) promote terminal differentiation of leukaemic promyelocytes, leading to complete remission in the majority of patients with APL and rapid resolution of the coagulopathy usually within 48 h, and a reduction in the early death rates. More latterly, arsenic compounds have been shown to be effective in the treatment of APL. They too, like ATRA, rapidly correct the bleeding syndrome, possibly by causing apoptosis of the leukaemic cells.

Antifibrinolytic agents

Tranexamic acid (TA) and aminocaproic acid (EACA) are synthetic antifibrinolytic agents. They act by blocking the lysine-binding sites of plasminogen, inhibiting the conversion of plasminogen into plasmin by tissue plasminogen

Table 12.6 Tranexamic acid use in bleeding

For local or generalized haemorrhage: Suggested dose 1 g t.d.s P.O.
For oral bleeding: 1 g as a mouthwash q.d.s.

activator. This will lead to decreased lysis of fibrin clots. In theory they are best used when bleeding is secondary to hyperfibrinolysis. *In vitro* studies have shown TA to be 10 times more potent and have a longer half-life than EACA. Within the United Kingdom EACA is rarely available and seldom used.

TA works best in the management of bleeding associated with enhanced fibrinolysis and in thrombocytopenic patients. It can be administered intravenously or orally. The intravenous route requires an infusion over 1 h, three or four times a day. This is rarely practical in palliative medicine and the oral route is favoured. It may take at least 2 days before improvement is seen and at least 4 days before cessation of bleeding (see Table 12.6).

Massive terminal haemorrhage

Massive terminal haemorrhage is defined as a major arterial haemorrhage from a patient in whom active treatment is not appropriate or possible, and which will inevitably cause death in minutes. It is usually associated with tumour erosion into the aorta or pulmonary artery (causing haematemesis or haemoptysis) or carotid or femoral artery (causing external bleeding). If a massive haemorrhage is unexpected, the only appropriate management may be to stay with the patient and attempt to comfort any distress.

Major haemorrhage may be preceded by smaller bleeds. Patients may have been receiving platelets and blood products, which have now been discontinued. If major haemorrhage is anticipated, an IV cannula should be inserted and appropriate drugs, already drawn up in a syringe, kept available at the bedside. Blue or green towels (which mask the colour of blood) should be available to help control the spread of blood.

In the event of a massive bleed, the aim of treatment will be to sedate rapidly and relieve patient distress from what will, by definition, be the terminal event. Where possible drugs should be given IV or else by deep IM injection.

Drug options

For summary see Table 12.7.

Table 12.7 Drugs used in massive terminal haemorrhage

Midazolam:	10–20 mg IV/IM
Ketamine:	150–250 mg IV or 500 mg IM
Diamorphine:	dose will vary

Midazolam

Midazolam 10 mg will sedate most patients. Heavy alcohol drinkers and patients on regular benzodiazepines may require larger doses. If the IV route is not available, the large volumes needed may be impractical.

Ketamine

The effect of ketamine is more predictable in palliative-care patients than benzodiazepines and opioids, since the patient is unlikely to have been taking it regularly, 150–250 mg ketamine IV will rapidly sedate a patient dying from a terminal haemorrhage. If the IM route is required; a larger dose of 500 mg will be required.

Opioids

These are less useful for the management of terminal haemorrhage for the following reasons.

(1) as a controlled drug, checking the drug out of the cupboard will hinder rapid access;

(2) diamorphine needs to be dissolved, leading to further delay;

(3) variable dose will be required depending upon how opioid-naïve the patient may be.

Editor's note: Ketamine may be difficult to obtain outside specialist units. Morphine and midazolam would be the standard options.

Conclusion

Thrombotic and bleeding complications of haematological malignancy are common at the end of life but may often be aggressively managed. The team should never lose focus on the issues that are important to the patient's quality of life, whilst supporting haemostatic and thrombotic defects. In the same way that a terminally ill patient's clinical condition will change from day to day, so we too must be comfortable in reviewing and altering our management of symptoms on a regular basis. There is no second chance to improve the quality of life of the dying patient.

References

1 Levitan, N. *et al.* (1999). Rates of initial and recurrent thromboembolic disease among patients with those without malignancy. Risk analysis using Medicare claims data. *Medicine* **78**, 285–291.

2 Johnson, M. J., Sproule, M. W., and Paul, J. (1999). The prevalence and associated variables of deep venous thrombosis in patients with advanced cancer. *Clin. Oncol* **11**, 105–10.

3 Weitz, J. I. (1997). Low molecular weight heparins. *N Eng J Med* **337**, 688–698.

4 Levine, M. and Lee, A. (2001). Treatment of venous thrombo-embolism in the cancer patient. *Acta Haematol* **106**, 81–87.

5 Palareti, G., Legnani, C., Lee, A. *et al.* (2000). A comparison of the safety and efficacy of oral anticoagulation for the treatment of venous thrombo-embolism in patients with or without malignancy. *Thromb Haemost* **84**, 805–810.

6 Johnson, M. J. (1997). Problems of anticoagulation within a palliative care setting: an audit of hospice patients taking warfarin. *Pall Med* **9**, 294–301.

7 Cowling, M. G. (1998). Filters inserted into the vena cava may be indicated may be useful for some indications. *Br Med J* **316**, 1830.

8 Bern, M. M., Lokich, J. J., Wallach, S. R. *et al.* (1990). Very low doses of warfarin can prevent thrombosis in central venous catheters: a randomized prospective trial. *Ann Intern Med* **112**, 423–428.

9 Monreal, M., Alastrue, A., Rull, M. *et al.* (1996). Upper extremity deep venous thrombosis in cancer patients with venous access decises-prophylaxis with a low molecular weight heparin (Fragmin). *Thromb Haemost* **75**, 251–253.

10 Degos, L. (ed.) (2001). Acute promyelocytic leukaemia. *Sem Haematol* **38**, 1–92.

Chapter 13

The management of sweating

Mary Miller

Introduction

Sweating is an uncommon but troublesome symptom in patients with advanced cancer. The key to successful management lies in establishing a diagnosis of the cause. This chapter discusses environmental and pharmacological measures to help manage the symptom.

Evidence to support the various management strategies outlined below is drawn from clinical practice and from trials, the majority of which are prospective. A minority are randomized and double-blind. Most trials have a small sample size, often less than 25 patients.

Sweating is the secretion of fluid, mainly water and sodium chloride, from the sweat glands onto the surface of the skin. Sweating (synonym: diaphoresis), a component of insensible water loss, occurs at rest as a normal physiological response to maintain homeostasis. The rate of sweating increases to compensate for an increase in body temperature. Evaporation of sweat aids cooling by convection of heat from the skin surface.

Physiology

Subcutaneous eccrine glands produce sweat. Cholinergic post-ganglionic sympathetic nerves innervate eccrine glands that are distributed over the surface of the body, except for the palms and the soles of the feet. Those eccrine glands that are situated on the palms, the soles of the feet and the axillae are under adrenergic control, and are stimulated in response to emotion.

Excessive sweating

Hyperhydrosis is the inappropriate production of large volumes of sweat. It is useful to record the severity of the symptom, and to monitor the effect of treatment. The tools that have been used include a six point scale (0 = no distress, 5 = severe distress)[1] and three grades of severity (see Table 13.1).[2]

Table 13.1 Severity of sweating

Mild sweating: no change of clothing necessary, symptom only reported after specific questioning.
Moderate sweating: no change of clothing necessary, washing of affected areas required, symptom volunteered by patient as a specific problem.
Severe sweating: symptom volunteered by patient and reported as drenching sweats, requiring a change of clothes, bed linen or both.

Prevalence

The prevalence of sweating has been reported to range from 0 to 16% in prospective studies of patients with advanced cancer. Interest in the symptom, the population studied, and publication bias may have contributed to a reported prevalence of one in six patients suffering from troublesome sweating. Clinical practice suggests a lower figure.

Patients with:

◆ lymphoma

◆ widespread disease

◆ hepatic metastases

are more likely to suffer from sweating.

Frequent change of clothes and bed linen, extra laundry, maintenance of a cool environment, and the meaning of the symptom may be a considerable burden for patients and their families.

Aetiology of sweating

There are many causes of sweating in patients with advanced cancer (see Table 13.2). It is important to diagnose the cause of the symptom. Aetiology will guide management.

Patients with advanced cancer reporting moderate to severe sweating are most likely to be sweating due to:

◆ sepsis

◆ widespread disease

◆ sex hormone insufficiency due to cancer treatment.

Assessment

Establish the time of onset and any events that precipitated the troublesome sweating, e.g. surgery or medication change (see Table 13.2). Identify any factors that cause sweating, factors that bring relief, measures used to manage the

Table 13.2 Aetiology of sweating

1. Thermoregulation—response to an increase in ambient temperature, muscular activity and ingestion of food.
2. Weakness.
3. Sepsis.
4. Pain, e.g. myocardial infarction, vertebral collapse.
5. Fear and anxiety.
6. Sex hormone insufficiency secondary to the menopause.
7. Sex hormone insufficiency due to cancer treatment, e.g. anti-androgens, anti-oestrogens, gonadal ablation.
8. Medication, e.g. opioids, anti-depressants, ethanol.
9. Neoplasia, e.g. lymphoma, hepatic metastases, widespread metastases, renal cell carcinoma.
10. Para-neoplastic fever.
11. Metabolic derangement, e.g. hypoglycaemia, hyperthyroidism.
12. Neurological lesion, e.g. Pancoast's tumour invading the sympathetic chain, diabetic meuropathy, autonomic neuropathy.
13. Autoimmune disease.
14. Idiopathic hyperhydrosis.
15. Other.

symptom to date, and their success. Establish the extent of metastatic disease. Document the sites of sweating and the severity of the symptom (see Table 13.1).

A symptom diary (Fig. 13.1) completed by the patient on a daily basis will help monitor response to drug management or intervention.

Measure temperature for a 24–48 h period to assess whether fever is associated with sweating. Examine the patient as indicated, e.g. for hepatomegaly or evidence of Pancoast's tumour. Investigate, as appropriate, to establish the aetiology of the sweating.

Management

Management of sweating is directed to the underlying aetiology of the symptom with the use of general measures to achieve symptom control (see Table 13.3).

Fever and sweating secondary to sepsis

Treatment of the underlying infection will bring about resolution of sweating and fever. Paracetamol 1 g 6-hourly will help reduce fever, the hypothalamic set

Diary of sweating

Please tick the most appropriate box for each question every day

	Date							
On average how has your sweating been in the past 24 h?	Very severe							
	Severe							
	Moderate							
	Mild							
	None							
How much has your sweating troubled you in the past 24 h?	Unable to think of other matters							
	A great deal							
	Moderately							
	Very little							
	Not at all							
How satisfied are you with the treatment of your sweating?	Very satisfied							
	Satisfied							
	Not satisfied or dissatisfied							
	Dissatisfied							
	Very dissatisfied							
How many changes of clothes (due to sweating) have been necessary in the past 24 h?								

Fig. 13.1 Symptom diary.

Table 13.3 Management of sweating

Treatment of the cause	plus	General management
Fever		
— sepsis		Environmental measures
— paraneoplastic		Pharmacological measures
Sex hormone insufficiency due to cancer treatment		
Other causes		

point being re-adjusted to a lower setting, while awaiting control of the infection. Sweating may increase to aid cooling of the body. It is not always appropriate to treat an infection in a patient with advanced cancer, which may have arisen as a consequence of the process of dying, e.g. pneumonia due to hypostasis.

Para neoplastic fever

In 5% of tumours, fever and sweating are not associated with an underlying infection. Release of 'pyrogens' from, or by, the tumour stimulates the temperature control centre in the hypothalmus causing pyrexia. Sweating occurs to aid cooling as the pyrexia abates. It is postulated that 'pyrogens' act via interleukin-6 and prostaglandins.

Pharmacological treatment of fever

Naproxen is the non-steroidal anti-inflammatory drug (NSAID) of choice in the management of para neoplastic fever and sweating. Complete resolution of symptoms was achieved in 90% of patients within 8 h.[3,4] The majority of patients responded to naproxen 250 mg b.d., some required 375 mg b.d.. The duration of effect was approximately one month. In cases of relapse, an alternative non-selective NSAID, diclofenac 25 mg t.d.s. or indomethacin 25 mg t.d.s., was effective. Symptom control was recaptured for a further month.

Corticosteroids will suppress fever and sweating due to infection or that occurring as a para neoplastic phenomenon, suggesting a different mechanism of action from NSAIDs, which have no effect on fever due to infection. Of patients, who were not receiving NSAIDs but who had a para neoplastic fever, 15% had complete resolution of symptoms with corticosteroids.[4] Doses of corticosteroids used varied considerably and effect persisted for the duration of treatment. A dose of dexamethasone 4 mg daily is a sensible starting point. The dose should be maintained at the lowest possible that achieves symptom control.

Sex hormone insufficiency due to cancer treatment

Sex hormone insufficiency due to cancer treatment may arise in several ways (see Table 13.4), leading to an acute onset of menopausal symptoms that is

Table 13.4 Aetiology of sex hormone insufficiency due to cancer treatment

Oophorectomy.

Orchidectomy.

Alkylating agent (chemotherapy) causing gonadal damage.

Anti-androgens (used in the management of prostate cancer).

Anti-oestrogens (used in the management of breast cancer).

Aromatase inhibitors (used in the management of breast cancer, prevent conversion of androgens to oestrogen in the peripheral tissue).

Gonaderolin analogue (used in the management of prostate cancer, depresses luteinising hormone production).

troublesome for a proportion of patients. The natural history is that symptoms will abate over the following months. Treatment is indicated if symptoms are troublesome. Medication used will need review after three to six months.

In men experiencing menopausal symptoms of sweating and hot flushes, diethylstilbestrol 1–3 mg daily, an oestrogen, helped alleviate symptoms in 75% of patients with prostatic cancer. Progestogens, medroxyprogesterone acetate 100–500 mg daily, or megestrol acetate 40–160 mg daily, may also be used, although there is little evidence available in the literature to support their use in the management of sweating. Cyproterone acetate's main mechanism of action is androgen blockade and it might therefore be expected to cause menopausal symptoms. Data from a single study has shown relief of menopausal symptoms. The authors postulate that relief occurred via the progestagenic action of cyproterone. Data from this single study should be interpreted with caution.

For women experiencing menopausal symptoms due to cancer treatment, progestogens are the only drug treatment available. Doses used are given above. Dietary approaches to managing symptoms are not covered here.

Other causes

Management is directed to the underlying aetiology if possible, e.g. treatment of fear, acute pain, or hyperthyroidism. Specialist advice should be sought in some situations, e.g. from dermatology colleagues in the management of idiopathic hyperhydrosis.

Environmental measures

These measures are appropriate regardless of the underlying aetiology. They include

- a reduction in the ambient temperature
- increased ventilation of the room
- the use of a fan.

Clothing and bedlinen

Cotton has a higher wicking ability and retains more moisture than synthetic fibres. Patient usually prefer to wear cotton. There is, however, insufficient evidence to guide choice of fibre in patients with advanced cancer.

It is best to avoid the use of plastic covers to protect pillows and bedding, if possible. Plastic prevents wicking of sweat away from the body surface. The body is less able to cool by evaporating sweat similar to the situation that occurs when there is high environmental humidity.

Help with laundry may greatly ease the burden for the patient and carers.

Pharmacological measures

These measures should be considered when the diagnosis of the cause of the sweating is unclear, where management directed to the correct diagnosis has failed to alleviate the symptom or while there is a delay before correction of the underlying diagnosis. The following order of drug use is suggested based on the volume of experience with the drug in managing the symptom of sweating balanced against the adverse effect profile of the drug.

Propantheline

Propantheline is an anti-muscarinic agent that decreases the rate of sweat secretion. There is considerable experience of it use in the management of idiopathic hyperhydrosis and to a lesser extent in the management of gustatory sweating as a complication of diabetic neuropathy. It is advisable to start at a dose of 15 mg once or twice daily increasing to 15 mg tds and 30 mg *nocte*. The dose may be increased to a maximum of 120 mg daily. In practice, adverse effects are too troublesome in patients with advanced cancer to achieve a maximum dose.

Thalidomide

The suggested mechanism of action of thalidomide is by suppression of tumour necrosis factor-alpha 100 mg *nocte* brought about a marked reduction in distress in 70% of patients.[1] Nausea and drowsiness were reasons for discontinuing the drug given by the other 30% of patients. Careful discussion is necessary with the patient and their carers before commencing thalidomide. Three patients refused to take part in the trial because of fears regarding thalidomide.

Clonidine

Clonidine is a centrally acting anti-hypertensive drug that causes central thermo-regulatory inhibition. It has been used to manage menopausal symptoms of sweating and hot flushes, and in the management of idiopathic hyperhydrosis. A dose of 50 μg t.d.s. should be used initially, increasing every second or third day to a maximum of 1.2 mg/day. One author suggested using the majority of the total daily dose at bedtime to prevent daytime sedation. Abrupt discontinuation of the drug may lead to a hypertensive crisis!

There is no trial data available to guide or support management in patients with advanced cancer.

Others

A number of other drugs have been used to alleviate sweating. Thioridazine was useful but has been withdrawn (in the UK), except in the management of schizophrenia. While there is pharmacological rationale for the use of other drugs, experience suggests that these drugs are unlikely to be effective. Cimetidine, a H_2 receptor antagonist has been suggested to alleviate sweating associated with morphine. Propranolol and benzodiazepines have been used when anxiety is thought to play a part in sweating, some of the sweat glands being under adrenergic control.

References

1   Deaner, P. B. (2000). The use of thalidomide in the management of severe sweating in patients with advanced malignancy: trial report. *Palliat Med* **14**, 429–31.

2   Quigley, C. S. and Baines, M. (1997). Descriptive epidemiology of sweating in a hospice population. *J Palliat Care* **13**, 22–6.

3   Tsavaris, N., Zinelis, A., Karabelis, A. *et al.* (1990). A randomized trial of the effect of three non-steriodal anti-inflammatory agents in ameliorating cancer induced fever. *J Int Med* **228**, 451–5.

4   Chang, J. C. (1988). Antipyretic effect of naproxen and corticosteroids on neoplastic fever. *J Pain Sym Manage* **3**, 141–4.

5   Torch, E. M. (2000). Remission of facial and scalp hyperhydrosis with clonidine hydrochloride and topical aluminium chloride. *South Med J* **93**, 68–9.

Chapter 14

Home care for terminally ill haematology patients

Cathy Alban-Jones and Lorraine Moth

The decision to leave hospital

The decision to leave hospital often follows a decision to stop chemotherapy, or aggressive treatment of an infection. Once this decision has been made, there may only be days, or at most weeks, of life remaining for the patient and family to be together, and quality of life is the paramount concern.

Frequently the patient and family will have invested in and hoped for the success of treatment right up until the moment it stops, and they often feel desperate to get home to familiar surroundings as soon as possible. Some patients may have been in hospital for many weeks or even months.

Rapid discharge from hospital is essential in these situations, but must provide patients and their families with adequate support to prevent unnecessary emergency admissions to a hospital that may be many miles from home.

This chapter covers:

- how to find out if patient and family want to be discharged home, after the decision has been made to stop life-prolonging therapy
- practical advice on communication about difficult issues with patients and families at this time
- the problems of patients with advanced haematological malignancy
- how to plan a smooth discharge
- how to recognize risk factors associated with complicated bereavement.

Chapter 10 on transitions will also have ideas on different approaches at this time.

A flowchart outlining the steps of discharge planning, which may be photocopied and used, or adapted for your unit is shown in Fig. 14.1.

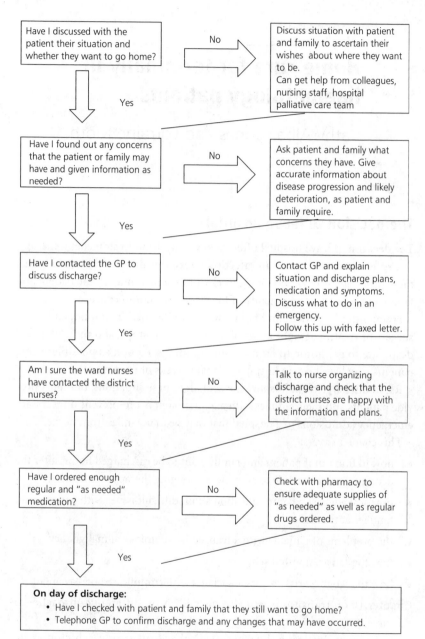

On day of discharge:
- Have I checked with patient and family that they still want to go home?
- Telephone GP to confirm discharge and any changes that may have occurred.

GP = General practitioner/family physician
district nurses = community nurses

Fig. 14.1 The steps of discharge planning.

Communication guidelines

Unlike other malignancies, once active treatment is stopped in haematology patients, their life-expectancy may only be days, or at best weeks. Staff working on the ward will often have developed a close relationship with the patient and family, and so be shocked and disappointed at the failure of treatment. This may make it difficult for them to explore with patients what they want at this tragic time. It is however, essential that this is done as it offers the patient and family the possibility of reclaiming dignity, hope, and a sense of control, when they may have had, inevitably, little or no control over their environment and treatment.

A terminal illness is often described as a 'hopeless situation', yet despairing attitudes about the effectiveness of treatment, or about the person's ability to respond to the knowledge of impending death, may mean that awareness of the relief of distressing symptoms is not fully explored, and that communication with the patient, family, and healthcare professionals is blocked. It is important to maintain the delicate balance between realistic hope and acceptance of the inevitable terminal care. Dying people and their relatives need encouragement to believe that symptoms can be alleviated, even when the disease is no longer curable, that dignity can be maintained, and that they themselves will have the courage, as well as support from professionals, to enable them to cope with a crisis. It is therefore essential to achieve an atmosphere of trust between the patient, their relatives, and healthcare professionals. When people are given misleading information, or when information is withheld from them, they often reach their own conclusions about the true state of affairs from what their bodies are telling them and from their reflections on what has been said. Total truth may not be helpful either, since emphasizing the terminal nature of the illness, and not the care and treatment that are still available, may drive dying people and their relatives to complete despair.

Prior to discharge it is important to allow patients and families the opportunity to discuss any fears or anxieties they may have. Good communication can take a great deal of time. Patients and relatives need to know that we as professionals are prepared to give them the time that they need. It is essential that professionals sit down in an unhurried manner at the patient's bedside, or in a quiet place, and allow eye-to-eye contact to occur. Privacy is equally important, as few people will risk talking about things as intimate and potentially distressing as fears about their illness, and dying, in the middle of a busy ward or clinic. When information of a medical nature is imparted to patients/relatives, it is always possible to adjust the mode of explanation to their individual knowledge and ability to understand. Information needs to be given gradually, allowing them time to mull over, absorb, and raise questions about one aspect before moving on to the next. It may be necessary to reiterate the information given several times. Often it is doctors who provide the information, while nurses can continue to clarify, interpret and expand on the facts given.

When you need to have such a conversation, make sure you have clarified all the facts before you embark on it. It is usually best to go with the nurse/doctor who is looking after that patient or with a specialist nurse who has been closely involved. Take the notes with you and if you have a bleep, give it to a colleague or the ward clerk or a secretary to answer until you have finished, and ask them to call you only if there is an emergency. If you cannot stay beyond a certain point, but your colleague who is also involved can stay longer, make that clear at the beginning of the discussion. Talk to your colleague before going in about the aims of the conversation, who is going to talk first, what you will do if you run into trouble, etc., and how you will solicit the patient's and family's agenda. Remember that they may be different.

You will always achieve more and run into fewer problems if you have a plan before you start, although you must be flexible and able to change tack if the situation demands this.

If possible, try and get a clinician involved in the discussion who knows the family and patient at least a little—trust is so important. Unfortunately, at weekends and in the evenings and nights, you may sometimes find that you have to talk to someone that neither you nor the ward nurse has met before. Acknowledge that this is not what you would wish when you introduce yourself but clarify that it is unavoidable on this occasion. Summarize the knowledge that you do have, e.g. that you have read the notes, heard about the patient at the team meeting or ward round, discussed everything with the consultant, GP or specialist nurse who knows the patient well.

Do not avoid the conversation because you are unsure how to approach it.

If you are inexperienced or unsure, you can help yourself and the family by:

◆ seeking advice from a senior colleague—even if they are unable to come to the ward, you can discuss it with them over the phone

◆ find a multidisciplinary approach—most commonly doctors and nurses will lead these conversations; if someone else has got to know the family well, involve them, even if you can only get phone advice

- do not wait for the perfect team to be assembled—this needs to be done fast as arrangements often take hours and more often a day or more to set up
- the hospital palliative care team (HPCT), who may have been involved, would expect to help out at this time
- the palliative care team can also be used for advice, even if the patient is not known to them or does not wish to be seen by them.

When discussing plans for the patient's discharge home from hospital, it is important to remember that different patients and families have different needs:

- some will require repeated short conversations and to be kept in touch with how plans for discharge are proceeding
- some will want only the barest information and not like to be reminded of the nearness of death
- some will not appear to acknowledge what is happening—this is less common in haematology patients (but not everyone wants to face death and it is not our job to force this on them).

In all conversations it is important to give truthful and accurate information, allowing time for questions and for patients and families to raise their concerns. It is the task of the healthcare professional to ensure that the family understands the gravity of the situation.

Communication with patient and family prior to discharge from hospital

In the planning of care and agreeing a management plan, patients need the opportunity to express their wishes and these are at the centre of all plans. Fears or religious concerns need to be explored and addressed appropriately, and respect given to cultural differences.

Patients can make valid choices only if they know:

- what is happening
- what help is available
- what is likely to, or may, happen in the future.

Families and carers will require the same information if they are to care for the patient who chooses to die at home.

Patients, families and carers need to know:

1. Information about the disease, expected events, and likely prognosis. The length of prognosis may significantly influence a family's ability to cope. When death is imminent, families are often able to 'pull out all the stops'

and draw on their own resources in order to cope with the situation. Over a period of time, however, these resources may become exhausted. It is always better to plan for a prolonged period, even when this is unlikely.

2. What support is available to them, and whom they should contact should a problem arise at any time of the day or night.

3. What changes to expect as the patient's condition deteriorates. Patients and families benefit from clear and concise information, and are less likely to be unnecessarily upset if they know what might happen.

Many people have not seen someone die, or even seen someone after death, and it is often very helpful to explain to relatives some details of the physical changes that may take place as their relative deteriorates—the sort of changes that clinicians will take for granted but which may be very frightening. For example:

♦   Changes in colour as death approaches like flushing with pyrexia, mottling of the skin as the circulation slows, cyanosis with hypoxia.

♦   Changes in breathing pattern—such as Cheyne–Stokes respiration.

♦   Noisy secretions. Families need to be reassured that, although this is often distressing for them to hear, patients are usually unaware that this is happening, and medication can be given to relieve the symptom.

♦   Lapse into semi/unconsciousness. Even though patients may not be able to respond, families need to know that often they can still hear, and that familiar noises will provide comfort to the patient.

♦   Immediately prior to this deterioration patients may become restless and/or agitated; even patients who have been moribund can experience restlessness and look unsettled. Relatives will need reassurance that this symptom can be controlled with medication and is part of the process of dying.

♦   If a patient is at risk of haemorrhage, relatives will need to know this. Discussion needs to include:
    •   any preconceived ideas they might have about what might happen;
    •   practical measures that they can take in the event of a haemorrhage;
    •   an action plan should the event occur.

♦   That death occurs when breathing stops. It is important for relatives to know that following the patient's death:
    •   there is no hurry to do anything
    •   they can touch and hold the patient, if they wish
    •   they can spend as much time with the patient as they wish

- they can prepare or help prepare the body for the undertakers
- they can keep the body at home before the funeral, if they wish
- they can contact a GP when the time feels right to certify the death.

Providing this information is given in a caring and sensitive manner, tailored to the relatives' needs, a great many fears and anxieties may be be relieved.

On a practical level, there is much that relatives can do to prepare their home for the patient's discharge from hospital. There is often much that the family can do to modify the home. This may include:

- moving the patient's bedroom downstairs where possible, so that access to, or sight of, the garden, or world outside, is possible
- placing favourite pictures where they can be easily seen
- flowers are a source of beauty and comfort for many patients who may not have been allowed them in hospital due to the risk of infection
- music, radio, and television can be placed within easy reach of the patient's bed or chair
- pets can offer companionship and love
- informality is the aim in creating a relaxed and loving environment where the patient feels supported and 'at home'.

Families may need to be given permission to maintain close physical contact with the patient. They may have been frightened of giving the patient an infection during intensive treatment. Much comfort can be derived from this both for the patient and for the family.

Visitors can be invited now, whereas they may not have been allowed (due to infection risk) or able to visit before. It may also be important to support people who want to restrict visitors, or to warn visitors that they may have to leave after a very short while, or even have to cancel their visit at the last moment. It is important that the patient and family have the freedom to do what they choose in these last days, which may even be looked back on as a very happy time.

Communication between professional teams

Patients may not have had very much contact with their GP since diagnosis, as their care is usually 'hospital focused', with any complications or blood support being dealt with by either their local hospital or the haematology centre where they are having treatment. It is therefore essential that the GP has an up-to-date summary of the patient's health status from the doctor/consultant in charge of the patient's care. Initially verbal contact should be made, followed by a faxed discharge summary. The following information needs should be provided:

1. The patients current health status and specific symptoms.
2. Plan of care. It needs to be made clear that the patient is for palliative/terminal care and that treatment is aimed at symptom control and improving quality of life.
3. Patients' and families' knowledge and level of understanding, together with a clear indication of the patients wish to die at home.
4. Action to take in the event of a medical emergency. Most medical emergencies in the last 48 h are irreversible, and treatment should be aimed at the urgent relief of any distress and concurrent symptoms. Drugs need to be made available for immediate administration in the home by community nursing staff without further consultation with a doctor. Directions regarding the use of such drugs needs to be written clearly and unambiguously. Therefore the drugs to be used should be discussed with the family doctor and community nurses, and preferably supplied by the hospital for the patient and family to take home—an emergency could happen the night that the patient is discharged.
5. A list of the patient's current medication and advice on breakthrough or 'as needed' medication. It is important to review medication prior to discharge with regard to need and route of administration. Previously 'essential' drugs are often no longer needed, although sometimes antibiotics are continued to ensure that the patient gets home to fulfil their wish of dying at home.
6. Estimated prognosis of the patient.
7. Date of next planned visit of GP or community nurses, in order to keep the patient and family informed.
8. A contact number(s) should be provided in the event that the GP needs to seek advice—remember this may be needed at any time, on any day of the week.
9. A copy of the discharge summary should be put in the patient's hospital notes.

Verbal communication between hospital and community nurses will also need to take place before the patient is discharged home. A discharge summary should then be written and given to the patient to give to the district nurse on her first visit. The information needs to be a comprehensive account of:

1. Nursing care required including dressings, pressure-area care, and any other specific nursing needs.

2. Information regarding the patient's and family's insight about what is happening, and a clear indication of the patient's wish to die at home.

3. A comprehensive assessment of the patient's physical, psychosocial, emotional, and spiritual needs.

4. Future care plan, including advice on what to do in the event of a medical emergency.

5. List of current regular and 'as needed' medication.

6. Knowledge of other care being provided, i.e. Marie Curie, Macmillan Nurses, Hospice at Home Teams. Sometimes the district will wish to make contact with any other available community services, as they work with them frequently.

If time allows, a home assessment by the occupational therapist will enable the provision of equipment that may be necessary to have at home for the comfort of the patient. Given that speed is often essential with haematology patients, it may be that the patient is discharged with basic aids only—the rest can follow as soon as possible. These will need to be prioritized by the hospital and should include items such as a commode, pressure-relieving aids/mattress, and urinals. If there is time, items such as a hospital bed are preferable, but should not delay discharge if a patient wants to die at home.

What services are available?

Figure 14.2 shows the services that may be involved in supporting a terminally ill patient at home.

Such services will vary from country to country and from area to area within the same country. Many of the teams available to look after patients at home are provided by voluntary or charitable organizations. In some countries, families and friends will provide the only support apart from a family doctor who may visit at home. The services described in Fig. 14.2 are variably available across the UK.

Symptom management in advanced haematological malignancy

Most difficult symptoms should be controlled before the patient leaves hospital but sometimes new ones will develop in the terminal phase or patients will prefer to get out of hospital before, for example, their pain is perfectly controlled. In this section, general guidance is given on those symptoms that may arise or need treatment after the patient has left hospital. Chapters 8 and 15 may also be helpful to consult.

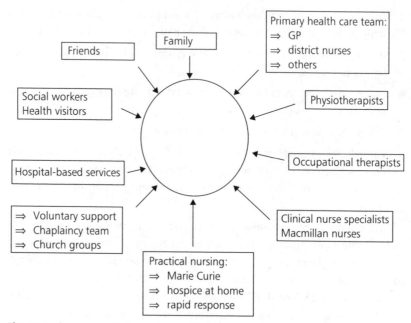

Fig. 14.2 The services that may be involved in supporting a terminally ill patient at home.

In this phase, maintaining or improving the patient's and the family's quality of life is paramount, and the risk/benefit for drugs may shift. Although unpleasant or uncomfortable adverse effects of drugs will still be unacceptable, the use of drugs or drug regimens which may potentially, though not inevitably, shorten life may be used.

Route of administration

Drugs should be given by mouth as long as possible. When the patient is dying, most drugs will be withdrawn. If analgesic, sedative, or anti-emetic drugs are needed when the patient cannot take oral medication, then a continuous subcutaneous infusion will be the method of first choice. The syringe driver can be loaded each day (or as needed) by the district nurse.

It is also possible for patient to be discharged with epidural infusions, depending on local regulations and expertise.

Many community teams are very committed to getting their patients home and will put in much extra work to achieve this.

General points about pain relief in the terminal phase

Bony pain is common in patients with leukaemia and myeloma

- Non-steroidals may have been contra-indicated due to low platelets or renal failure. When the patient is dying, this risk may become acceptable to them. It is an individual decision that can only be made after careful but frank discussion.

- Analgesia needs to be titrated, using the WHO ladder, until adequate pain relief is achieved.

- Palliative radiotherapy can be helpful in relieving pain caused by bony deposits from myeloma and it may be worth delaying discharge for one day if this is indicated. New crush fractures may occur after discharge and then management will depend on the individual circumstances of the patient. Such decisions include whether it is worth going back for another fraction of radiotherapy as a day patient or whether the journey would be too difficult.

Patients with lymphoma

Further tumour growth or increasing lymphadenopathy causing pain may develop after discharge. It is important to remember that:

- many patients with advanced cancer have more than one pain

- patients can develop novel neuropathic pain once discharged, especially as their tumour masses enlarge

- oral morphine solution (or other strong opioids like oxycodone, fentanyl, or hydromorphone) are usually effective in relieving the visceral component of pain

- neuropathic pain is usually poorly responsive or only partially responsive to opioids and will need alternative pharmacological therapy.

Nausea

It is frequently inappropriate or impossible to reverse the cause of nausea in the terminal phase. Some examples include:

- hypercalcaemia
- renal failure
- raised intra-cranial pressure
- bowel obstruction.

It may be possible, however, to stop some drugs that may be exacerbating nausea, and sometimes fear or anxiety about what is happening may need specific help.

Other therapeutic measures to relieve nausea, which may be considered and easily used at home, are

◆ massage

◆ relaxation

◆ aromatherapy

◆ acupuncture, where underlying condition allows.

Massage and relaxation are especially helpful if nausea is related to anxiety or fear. Relatives can be taught how to do simple hand or foot massage, and breathing exercises for relaxation. Ginger has been shown to relieve nausea and may be taken in the form of capsules or by taking foods containing ginger.

Thrombocytopenia

Many haematology patients will have very low platelets at the end of their lives and will be at risk of bleeding. By adhering to a few simple rules, the risk of bleeding can be reduced:

◆ taking care when turning patients will reduce bleeding and bruising;

◆ nursing patients on a soft, pressure-relieving mattress will also be beneficial and promote comfort;

◆ vigilance with mouth care (see below) will help prevent bleeding from gums; tranexamic acid (500 mg t.d.s. to 1.5 mg q.d.s.) may be given to reduce the possibility of a surface bleed providing DIC is not suspected;

◆ if bleeding is from a pressure sore or open wound, using haemostatic dressings such as kaltostat may help.

Major bleeds

One of the most distressing events that can happen to a patient with low platelets is a major bleed, which is a terminal event. Families need to be warned about the possibility of this happening in a calm and constructive way, so that they are able to explore their fears about this and have an action plan should this event arise, including emergency contact numbers of their GP, district nurse, and any other agency that could help them. It should also be stressed that while this event may happen, it is not common.

A major bleed may be external or internal—the patient will become shocked, clammy, and cold.

If the bleed is external, having coloured towels to hand will help to cover the site of bleeding and also mask the extent of the blood loss. If the patient is at home and there is no nurse (e.g. Marie Curie) present, the family will need to contact the GP or district nurses as an emergency.

Having a syringe preloaded with midazolam 10–20 mg +/− diamorphine ready at home will save time when they arrive. Sublingual lorazepam 1 mg or diazepam, 10–20 mg, per rectum, could be given by the family while they are waiting, if they feel confident enough to do so. Staying with the patient is important in order to reduce the patient's anxiety and also that of their family.

Pyrexia

Haematology patients are taught the importance of taking their temperature and rushing to hospital if their temperature is raised, from the beginning of their treatment. Thus it is very difficult for patients and their families when treatment is stopped, to relax those guidelines that they have lived by for so long, and to accept treating pyrexia symptomatically and not with intravenous drugs. This needs to be borne in mind when providing care for such patients and families.

An infection or the disease itself may cause high and fluctuating temperatures. Pyrexia may also be accompanied by sweating. Both symptoms are distressing for patients and can often be minimized using a few simple guidelines:

◆ paracetamol, either orally or rectally, will help reduce pyrexia
◆ using a fan to keep the room cool and air circulating will help
◆ sweating may be relieved by naproxen.

If your patient is unable to tolerate NSAIDs due to low platelets and increased risk of bleeding use an alternative drug such as

◆ amitriptyline 25–50 mg at night
◆ probantheline 15–30 mg every 8 h
◆ propranolol 10–20 mg every 8 h.

Again, keeping the air temperature cool and avoiding synthetic fibres in clothing and bedding may help.

The experience of being unable to breathe easily leads to fear and anxiety, making breathing even more difficult. Where appropriate, treatment of the underlying cause of breathlessness should be considered. The following interventions may also help:

◆ a small dose of oral morphine, i.e. 2.5–5 mg liquid oral morphine, given as needed, can help reduce breathlessness in many patients
◆ this may be combined with an anxiolytic, especially at night, so that patients are able to have a reasonable period of sleep

- keeping the air around the mouth and nose moving by using a hand-held fan reduces the experience of breathlessness and is something patients can do for themselves
- teaching breathing exercises using abdominal breathing techniques has also been shown to be beneficial
- some patients, especially those with hypoxaemia, may benefit from oxygen given via nasal cannulae or by mask which ever is preferred.

Pruritus

Unrelieved itching inhibits sleep and is exhausting for patients.

- Simple measures such as maintaining a cool environment and cooling the skin may help.
- Antihistamines can help to reduce itching and may also help promote sleep.
- Creams, such as aqueous cream/menthol 1–20% are easily available from community pharmacists and can ease the discomfort caused by incessant itching.

Mouth care

Mouth care is an important part of caring for haematology patients when they are dying. The aims are:

- to prevent oral infection leading to a sore mouth
- to prevent bleeding from gums and teeth due to low platelets
- to keep the mouth moist and comfortable.

Regular mouth care using a soft toothbrush can prevent infections and a coated tongue, which can affect taste and enjoyment of any food or drink:

- using petroleum jelly on dry lips prevents cracking and soreness
- dry mouths can be relieved by sucking ice cubes or by using an artificial saliva spray such as glandosane
- if the tongue is coated, use effervescent vitamin C tablets, 250 mg q.d.s., which should be allowed to dissolve on the tongue, together with regular mouthwashes and oral care
- corsadyl is an effective mouthwash for general hygiene, while difflam is the mouthwash of choice when soreness is present, as it has an analgesic effect
- sucking pineapple has also shown to help relieve a coated tongue and is very refreshing for patients

- if a patient has severe mucositis, it may be necessary to use a diamorphine syringe driver to control the pain, together with morphine mouthwashes— the dose being titrated to the patients need
- oral candidiasis needs to be treated with a systemic antifungal agent (see Chapter 7).

Constipation and diarrhoea

If a patient has only days to live, interventions such as suppositories and enemas may not be appropriate because the discomfort caused may outweigh the possible good.

Skin care is very important if someone has diarrhoea, in order to prevent excoriation and breakdown of the skin. Gentle washing of the skin and the application of a barrier cream, such as sudocrem, after each episode of diarrhoea can help prevent deterioration in skin condition and soreness, and promote comfort for the patient.

Confusion/agitation

Reasons for confusion/agitation are many and include:

- hypoxia due to anaemia or chest disease
- renal failure causing uraemia
- hypercalcaemia (myeloma patients)
- drugs
- constipation
- infection
- a full bladder.

As with any other symptom, it is important to try and establish the cause of the confusion/agitation and, where appropriate, treat it.

It may be more important to make the diagnosis that the patient is dying.

It is not always possible to be certain in a dying patient and sometimes it may not be appropriate to keep looking. Even if a dying patient is hypoxic, reversing this may make little difference. It is only part of an inevitable process. It may be more important to talk to the family about what is happening and use symptom-control such as sedation:

- haloperidol, either orally or via a syringe driver, can be effective for confusion, especially where there is an element of paranoia
- midazolam is an anxiolytic, which can be very helpful for terminal agitation—it may be given via a syringe driver or intermittent SC injections
- tiny doses of 2.5–5 mg in 24 h (in the frail elderly or very weak) can give anxiolysis without sedation
- larger doses such as 30 mg in 24 h will generally sedate
- the usual maximum dose is around 90 mg but this is very infrequently used.

A patient who is dying, and who was on regular opioid therapy, will often obtain good symptom control with diamorphine (based on previous needs) and midazolam given by continuous subcutaneous infusion.

General measures, which can reduce agitation and confusion, are as follows:

- To keep the patient's environment quiet, with people who are familiar to him/her. Avoid any loud or sudden noise, which may increase any agitation.
- Explaining carefully any procedures calmly and in a language the patient can understand will help reduce agitation. Repeat the same words or simple phrase to explain what is happening to someone who is cognitively impaired, rather than giving the same information many different ways.
- During any periods of lucidity it is important to stress to the patient that the confusion is due to the disease, as they may fear that they are going mad or losing their grip on reality, which can be very frightening and increase any agitation.
- Families will need extra support at this time, as watching a loved relative being confused and possibly agitated is very distressing. An explanation to the family about what is causing the confusion and how they can best help the patient can help relieve their anxiety and feeling of helplessness.
- Using a dim night-light, big calendars and clocks can help keep people orientated.

Support before and after the patient's death

Support of patients and family should always be preceded by careful assessment of their expressed needs and concerns. This allows an individual and flexible approach to be adopted for each person.

In the hospital, the supportive relationship between healthcare professionals and a terminally ill person has a natural end when the person is discharged or dies. This is not always so. Members of the family may have grown very close and dependent on the ward team during the course of some years of treatment or during a very intense time. Occasionally it may be difficult for us to close contact with a person whom we have grown to like, and who may be grateful for the care received from us. However, it is important to allow the person to grow in independence, and it is necessary for our own emotional well-being that we do not see ourselves as the only people capable of giving such support. Any bereavement support should normally be given in the community or at least outside the unit, to enable the family to lose contact with the hospital and begin a different sort of life.

It is important, for everyone concerned to recognize that grief is a normal response to the death of a loved one and that everyone experiences grief in a different way. It is also important to recognize that staff feel grief too and we need to be able to understand this and seek the sort of support that helps.

There are many voluntary organizations such as CRUSE, who offer help to the grieving. The National Association of Bereavement Counsellors can put families in touch with a local bereavement counsellor if a family feel they need more formal counselling.

Further reading

Charles-Edwards, A. (1983). *The nursing care of the dying patient.* Oxford: Oxford University Press.

Clark, D. and Seymour, J. (1999). *Reflections on palliative care.* Oxford: Oxford University Press.

Field, D. (1989). *Nursing the dying.* Routledge.

Fredman, G. (1997). *Death talk.*

Hunt, R. (1997). Place of death of patients: choice versus constraint. *Prog Pall Care,* 5, 238–41.

Laussaniere, J. M. and Auzanneau, G. The quality of terminal care in haematology. *Eur J Pall Care,* 2 (4).

Lugtton, J. (1987). *Communicating with dying people and their relatives.* Austen Comish Publishers Ltd.

O'Neill, B. and Rodway, A. (1998). Care in the community. *BMJ,* 316, 31.

Chapter 15

The last days of life

Fiona Hicks

Introduction

Despite important advances in the treatment of haematological malignancies, many patients continue to die of their disease. When death becomes inevitable, patients, families and staff often struggle with the depth of sadness surrounding the event and clinical staff may feel profoundly inadequate at not being able to change the course of the illness. Although death cannot be averted, there is much that can be done to improve the last days of life for patients and their families. Memories made at this time are hard to dispel and often live with families and staff throughout their bereavement. Good terminal care is therefore not only important for the patient but helps to create positive memories for families and staff.

The key to good management in the last days of life is the recognition that death has become inevitable and the focus of care is changed. There are several texts that cover the management of the dying patient and general principles will not be repeated here. However, there are some aspects to terminal care in haematological oncology that pose particular problems:

- the terminal phase may be short following intensive treatment with curative intent
- palliation may require ongoing 'high-tech' interventions, which are invasive
- patients may be in a regional centre a long way from home
- patients are often young.

These issues and many others that relate particularly to this group of patients will be discussed in this chapter.

Evidence

There is little published research into the management of terminal care in haemato-oncology. This chapter is based on clinical experience, including

Proceedings from the First World Congress on Palliative Care in Haematology,[1] qualitative research on the views of bereaved relatives,[2] and published case reports.

Changing the focus of care

Patients with haematological malignancies fall into two broad groups at the end of life:

♦ those who die during the phase of active treatment

♦ those who die from advanced progressive disease.

Patients dying during active treatment

This is often the most difficult group of patients to manage, for staff and families alike. Death may be caused:

♦ directly by treatment-related toxicity

♦ by complications such as haemorrhage or infection

♦ by treatment failure.

The terminal phase is often short, with little time to prepare patients and families for subsequent events. Staff often feel a profound sense of failure or even guilt, particularly when patients and families have invested heavily in the hope of cure with the burdens of treatment being significant. Changing the goal of care in this situation takes courage and must be a decision that is accepted by the whole clinical team.

Patients who die of advanced, progressive disease

Patients in this category may have a more predictable terminal phase and a more gentle transition in the focus of care. However, supportive care with blood products and antibiotics can extend life for considerable periods and the decision that a patient is dying can prove very difficult (e.g. myelodysplastic syndromes). Again, all members of the clinical team should understand and agree with the transition point if good terminal care is to be achieved.

For both groups of patients, when death is approaching all interventions should be aimed towards comfort for the patient and open communication with family members. Treatment-related toxicity is not acceptable even in the short term, as there will be no long-term gain.[3] The recognition that death is approaching is a clinical skill that requires experience and can be particularly finely balanced in this population, but it is a necessary prerequisite to achieving good terminal care. For both groups of patients, the terminal phase may be short with little time for adjustment.

Facilitating choice

Although patients and families may feel that they had little choice but to accept the treatments offered during the curative or palliative phases of treatment, there are potentially several choices available for terminal care. Facilitating choice requires open and sensitive two-way communication, as well as an understanding of the services available for patients at this time. The provision of accurate information can enable families to make choices but may be difficult if there is uncertainty surrounding prognosis. Decisions will need to be made quickly if the situation is changing rapidly.

Place of care

Most patients and families will want to consider the place of care. The clinical team will need to have a good knowledge of services available in the community and of local hospice provision. For patients treated in regional centres, this may mean staff having a detailed knowledge of several community and hospice services across the region. Families will need some understanding of the implications of home care and the level of support that can be provided at home. Although hospices are expert at managing terminal care, for patients who have not had previous contact with hospice services, investing in new relationships at this time may prove difficult. Patients may elect to stay in hospital, being cared for by staff they have come to know, in familiar surroundings, either on a haematology ward or the bone marrow transplant unit. Although the physical environment of a hospital is rarely as appropriate as a hospice, and the training and focus of staff reflects the curative setting, familiarity may be important at a time when other things feel out of control.

Supporting the family

Changing gear from curative/life-prolonging therapy to terminal care, is clearly a stressful time for families. Some may not have contemplated the possibility of treatment failure, for others it is the confirmation of their worst fears. Powerful emotions may need to be held in check while they support the patient and other family members. Practical considerations and ethical dilemmas may seem overwhelming. Families need the time and space to be able to feel and express their grief, disappointment, anger, or resentment. Anger may be particularly strong for those who have invested heavily in the possibility of cure and although the odds of treatment failure may have been explained at the outset, they did not apply them to their own situation. Many families feel alienated by a 'high-tech' environment in hospital and this may be compounded by the care being given in a regional centre a long way from home, other family, and friends. Families need help to regain some control of the situation by expressing their pain and feeling able to make choices. Practical support may reduce some of the family stress, e.g. providing accommodation for close family members who live at a distance from the unit will make life significantly easier.

Other patients and families

Relatives often gain support from the families of other patients who they may have come to confide in over the months of illness and treatment. It is important for staff to acknowledge this as it may impact on the care needed by other patients and families over the period of terminal care and after a patient's death.

Involving children

Special consideration is needed for families with young children. Visiting may be difficult both in practical and emotional terms and must be handled with sensitivity. Families are often concerned that the patient's appearance has changed significantly, with cachexia, alopecia, bruising, bleeding of gums/nose, and intravenous lines. They would wish for children to remember their loved one as they were in health and not to be frightened by their current appearance. This must be balanced against the fear of the unknown, as children who are prevented from visiting may imagine that they are being kept away because they are in some way the cause of their parents' problem or even believe that their parent is being tortured or looking unimaginably horrific. Children often fantasize about what is happening if they are kept away, and their fantasies are unpredictable. Expert help may be needed to help families with young children to handle such a situation as parents are often struggling so much with their own grief that they cannot give it due consideration. Good nursing care can improve a patient's appearance and facilitate such visiting, which may be extremely important for each person in the moment, and also to those left behind in bereavement.

Supporting the staff

Supporting staff working in this area is vital to enable them to provide and continue to provide good care, and to maintain their own emotional health. In services that are often overstretched and understaffed, this is an area that is too often seen as a luxury and sacrificed in the face of clinical pressures. However, this work is not only technically demanding, it is also highly emotionally charged, and if this is neglected it will affect the quality of care. All seniorities of staff in all the professions in the clinical team should have the opportunity to reflect on:

• the care they offer to patients
• the effect this has on themselves when a patient dies.

This is particularly true when patients die on the bone marrow transplant unit, where staff have a prolonged and close interaction with patients who have tolerated highly toxic treatments with the hope of achieving a cure. Staff may feel guilty that they have shortened a patient's life, albeit with the best of intentions. This may cause dissent within the caring team, with some members questioning whether the patient ever really understood the implications of a bone marrow transplant. Team members may disagree about whether the patient is dying, and containing this within the clinical team is vital for the confidence of patients and families. There must be opportunities for staff to question each other and to express how they feel in the situation. This may need external facilitation and is best done as a regular multidisciplinary meeting that becomes part of the core business of the unit. The hospital palliative care team may be in a position to provide support in these matters.

The cure/care dilemma

Staff working in haematology often find it difficult to maintain the parallel strands of their role, with some patients receiving intensive therapy aimed at cure alongside patients who are dying. There is a cultural shift between the two elements of work, and passing from one room to the next while making such a shift can be a challenge. There may be a tension between some staff who would encourage dying patients and their families to move off the unit to go home or to a hospice or general ward, and other staff members who want to continue through terminal care to achieve a sense of completion. It takes significant self-awareness to be able to offer patients and families true choice in this situation.

Reviewing therapies

When changing the focus of care during the last days of life, staff must re-evaluate all aspects of the care they provide. Treatment should be aimed at comfort and a flexibility of care towards families encouraged.

Ward policies should be reviewed where possible, provided that this does not interfere with the care of other patients. Examples of this may be allowing flowers in a room despite the infection risk, or relaxing procedures around visiting.

Drugs should be stopped if they are not contributing to comfort, and interventions such as total parental nutrition, intravenous infusions, blood product support, blood tests, and regular observations should be re-evaluated. Patients and families may find this particularly difficult, and care is needed to prevent them feeling abandoned. For some patients, discontinuing interventions will need to be gradual and for all it should be accompanied by honest, sensitive communication.

Nursing observations may be discontinued but they must be replaced by more appropriate care such as spending time talking with patients and families. Mouth care and pressure-area care remain important for comfort.

Doctors may feel concern that part of their familiar role is less relevant but should not underestimate the importance of continuing to visit patients on ward rounds, even when the patient has become unconscious. Medical staff entering a room where an unconscious patient is surrounded by their family may feel at a loss as to what to say or that they are intruding on the family's grief. However, families find it comforting to know that the care continues and adjustments to medications for symptom management may be needed, in addition to the opportunity to answer families' questions. A simple introductory phrase, such as 'Do you think he is comfortable?' is often sufficient to encourage family members to express any concerns. Nursing colleagues also value the contribution of doctors in terminal care, as it maintains the team approach.

Supporting patients

The principles of symptom management, psychological, social and spiritual support can be applied to terminal care whatever the diagnosis.

Symptom management

The cause of death in haematology patients is usually bone marrow failure and good symptom management may require active support with blood products up to the time of death. Intravenous access is often present and can be used to deliver drugs required for comfort when the oral route is no longer practical. If the patient does not have IV access, parenteral drugs can be given via a subcutaneous syringe driver, even for patients with a reduced platelet count. If oozing around the needle becomes a problem, this may need to be reviewed. Analgesia delivered by transdermal patches may be an alternative, but most patients will require a combination of analgesic, anti-emetic and anti-secretory/sedative drugs, which are best delivered subcutaneously. Renal failure is a common feature in these patients and care is needed when prescribing drugs excreted by the kidney or those with active metabolites that are renally excreted. Although diamorphine remains the parenteral analgesic of choice, the dose may need to be reduced in this instance or an alternative such as alfentanyl prescribed, which does not have active metabolites excreted by the kidney.[4] Signs of diamorphine overdose in patients who have been receiving opioids for pain control for prolonged periods may be more subtle than repiratory depression and pin-point pupils. Patients may develop myoclonus, confusion, worsening emesis, or terminal agitation. Terminal restlessness describes the symptom complex in dying patients who appear to be in discomfort, either physically, emotionally, or spiritually. These patients will usually be semiconscious and unable to describe the source of their anguish. Attention must be given to possible contributing factors such as poor pain control, urinary retention, constipation, or accumulation of renally excreted drugs. If no reversible cause can be identified, the only course of action may be to sedate the patient to provide relief. Midazolam given subcutaneously or intravenously can be effective at doses ranging from 10 mg to 60 mg over 24 h. If the dying phase if prolonged, tachyphylaxis may occur, particularly in younger patients, and an alternative sedative such as phenobarbitone may be used.

Ethical issues

Ethical dilemmas in end-of-life care should be discussed within the multiprofessional clinical team in the hope of reaching a consensus decision. This is often an area where divisions within the team will come to the fore, and to maintain healthy team-working, external facilitation may be required. Some hospitals now have clinical ethics committees, which can be a valuable resource in difficult circumstances. For others, the hospital-based palliative care team may provide the facilitation required.

Resuscitation

Resuscitation status should not be a controversial issue at this stage of treatment, as it is clear that any attempt at resuscitation would be futile. This should be recorded clearly in the notes but there is no necessity to discuss it directly with the family. If communication has been effective with family members it should be clear that the goal of treatment is comfort and many families find it confusing if 'Do Not Attempt Resuscitation' orders are discussed with them. Indeed, some families are asked to comply with such orders, which can leave them bewildered by the aims of treatment and they carry an overwhelming burden that they may have shortened the life of a loved one by agreeing to the order. If families are asked to make a choice in this situation, they may feel that there is a real choice on offer, which clearly is not the case.

Withdrawing treatments

Decisions regarding the continuation of parenteral nutrition or intravenous fluids may be more finely balanced. It is important for staff and families to continue to focus all care towards patient comfort, and the emotive nature of nourishment and hydration means that families will often have to be encouraged to do this. The lack of any convincing research into the use of fluids to relieve thirst in terminal care, often makes this an individual choice. The balance between burdens and benefits of treatment will vary between individuals and for individuals as the disease progresses. The value of interventional treatment should be weighed against the fact that this may prevent patients from getting home to die and create a physical barrier between patients and families. Clinical staff may be tempted to focus care on the interventions rather than on aspects of care that are more important at this time.

Case study

A 77-year-old man had received haemodialysis for 2 years following the diagnosis of multiple myeloma with light chain nephropathy. His myeloma had been treated with chemotherapy and concurrent infections managed with intravenous antibiotics. However, his disease had become chemoresistant and he now required regular blood and platelet transfusions. He and his family had become very well known to the haematology and dialysis staff, who felt that he was becoming increasingly depressed, although this had not yet been treated. He had expressed a wish that it was 'all over' and that he could be in his own home. He developed resistant hypercalcaemia and a pyrexia with consequent delirium. His family wanted to take him home for terminal care, although it was not clear that they really understood how close to death he was without dialysis. Staff on the ward and in the dialysis unit were divided about what should be done:

- keep him in hospital to treat his pyrexia, continue dialysis and if his delirium improved, address his possible depression and explore what care he really wanted at this stage of his illness
- allow the family to take him home and arrange dialysis in a satellite unit close to home, although he may be too unwell to attend and this may be giving confusing messages to his family
- allow his family to take him home for terminal care, acknowledging that he will die of renal failure within a matter of days.

Resolving such issues within the caring teams who have become very close to the situation can be complex. All staff have their own views about end-of-life care, their own beliefs, and priorities. External facilitation can help to clarify the issues and bring focus to discussions, exploring the pros and cons of each option. Perhaps most important of all, acknowledging that there is no 'right' answer and ensuring that the team come to an understanding that any decision made is the best possible, on the information available, at that time. This should prevent staff blaming others if events turn out less well than expected.

The role of the hospital palliative care team

Referral

Timely referral to the hospital-based palliative care team (HPCT) is essential if it is to play a full role in the last days of a patient's life. The dilemma of when to refer to palliative care services is covered in Chapters 8 and 10; this is a particularly difficult issue for patients dying on active treatment. For patients undergoing bone marrow transplantation, for example, palliative care could be introduced when treatment options are first discussed alongside the risk of treatment failure. If patients and families have not been introduced to palliative care staff in advance of the terminal phase of care, sensitive introductions are necessary to prevent patients feeling rejected by staff they have come to know well. Some patients and families decline direct input, as it is too difficult to invest in new staff during such rapidly changing and distressing circumstances. In this situation, the HPCT can still provide support and advice to the ward staff who are directly involved in the care.

For patients with advancing disease who have been receiving active treatment with palliative intent for some time, palliative care staff can help in defining the transition point to terminal care. This task is made easier if a relationship has been previously established with the patient, but defining the point at which a transition to terminal care occurs remains difficult, and antibiotics and blood product support may be continued as symptomatic treatments.

Staff support

The HPCT can facilitate open communication where necessary within the haematology team, resolving disagreements about the focus of care and supporting staff in their bereavements. Haematology staff usually work in busy units and time for staff support is often sacrificed in the face of other clinical pressures. However, caring for dying patients inevitably affects medical and nursing staff, and quality of care is undermined in the long term if attention is not paid to this aspect of the work. Facilitating regular meetings, which become part of the ward culture, goes some way to helping in this area.

Symptom-management

Specialist palliative care services have considerable expertise in managing complex symptom problems at the end of life. They can provide advice based on a detailed knowledge of the pharmacology of drugs used at the end of life and their handling in organ failure. Suggestions for administering drugs by alternative routes to enable patients to get home more easily can be made, in addition to advice on aspects of nursing care.

Discharge planning

The hospital palliative care team will have a detailed knowledge of services, both in the community and in hospices, which can help families to decide on the most appropriate place of care. This is particularly important in regional centres who may have patients from several different areas, with varying service provision. Access to accurate and timely information is vital if a patient is to achieve a good discharge in a complex situation with rapidly changing needs.

More discussion will be found in Chapter 14.

Family support

Members of the palliative care team can provide families with the opportunity to express their anger or disappointment at the disease or treatment with staff who have not been directly involved in prescribing or administering therapy. The HPCT has not invested in potential cure in the same way as others and families may need to express emotion without the fear of letting the ward team down or compromising the treatment. Support to families can be extended into bereavement. Where families are concerned about young children, they can access specialist support both during the illness and through bereavement.

Concluding thoughts

Although death is rarely welcomed, and is almost universally a time of sadness, much can be done to alleviate some of the suffering and manage the situation successfully. This requires open communication, flexibility, clinical skill, and good team-working and can be achieved for patients dying of haematological malignancies.

References

1 Laussaniere, J. M. and Auzanneau, G. (1995). The quality of terminal care in haematology. *Eu J Pal Care* 2 (4), 169–172.
2 McGrath, P. (2002). End of life care for haematological malignancies: the technological imperative and palliative care. *J Pal Care* 18 (1), 39–47.
3 Ashby, M. and Stoffell, B. (1991). Therapeutic ratio and defined phases: proposal of ethical framework for palliative care. *BMJ* 302, 1322–1324.
4 Dickman, A., Littlewood, C., and Varga, J. (2002). Alfentanyl. In *The syringe driver*, p. 18. Oxford University Press.

Further reading

Twycross, R. and Lichter, I. (1998). The terminal phase. In *Oxford textbook of palliative medicine* (2nd edn), pp. 977–995. Oxford University Press.

Twycross, R., Wilcock, A., and Thorp, S. (1998). *Palliative care formulary.* Radcliffe Medical Press.

Woof, R., Carter, Y., Harrison, B. *et al.* (1998). Terminal care and dying. In *Handbook of palliative care* (ed., Faull, C., Carter, Y., Woof, R.), pp. 307–332. Blackwell Science.

Working Party on Clinical Guidelines in Palliative Care, National Council for Hospice and Specialist Palliative Care Services (1997). *Changing gear—guidelines for managing the last days of life in adults.*

Index

haematopoietic growth factors (HGFs) 85
haemolysis 181, 182
haemolytic uraemia syndrome 67, 205
haemorrhage
  acute leukaemias 40
  terminal 207–8, 230–1
  see also bleeding
haemostatic effects 191
haloperidol 122, 123, 131, 234
hand washing 36
Hasenclever prognostic score 15
heparin 195
heparin-like anticoagulants 204
hepatic complications 68
herpes simplex (HSV) 36, 66, 107–8
herpes zoster 36, 140
Hodgkin's disease 13, 14, 15–17, 24
home care 219–35
home modification 225
hope 171
hopelessness 132
hospital palliative care team 245–6
hydration 5
hydronephrosis 21
hyoscine butylbromide 123, 124
hypercalcaemia 24
hyperhydrosis, *see* sweating
hypersplenism 200
hyperviscosity 6
hypnosis 82

iatrogenic bleeding 205
illness, making sense of 166, 167
imipramine 144
impotence 26
infection
  acute leukaemias 33–7
  lymphoma 21–2
  mucosal injury 105–8
  myeloma 6
  stem cell transplantation 66, 69–70
infertility 26, 71
inguinal lymphadenopathy 20
insomnia 133–4
intra-spinal therapy 149
ionizing radiation 44
iron-deficiency anaemia 180,
    181, 182
iron overload 71
isolation 76
itching 13, 24, 232

ketamine 146–7, 208

lamotrigine 143
laser therapy 104
last days of life 41, 237–47
laxatives 125
leucopenia 26

leukaemias, acute 29–42
  diagnosis 29–32
  epidemiology 29–32
  gastro-intestinal complications 38–9
  haemorrhage 40
  infection 33–7
  last days of life 41
  lymphoblastic 29, 31–2
  management 33–9
  mouth care 36
  myeloblastic 29, 30–1, 32–3
  nutritional support 39–40
  palliative care 32–3
  prognosis 30
  promyelocytic 30–1, 206
  pulmonary complications 37–8
  renal dysfunction 39
  respiratory support 38
  stem cell transplantations 31, 32
  treatment 29–32
  vaccination 37
levomepromazine 123, 124
Lidoderm® 148
life worth living 171–2
lignocaine 145–6, 148
linear analogue scale assessment (LASA) 178
local anaesthetics 99–100, 145–6
low molecular weight heparin 195
lymphadenopathy 19–20
lymphoma 11–27
  anaemia 21
  Ann Arbor staging 14
  bleeding risk 22
  bone marrow failure 21–2
  bowel obstruction 20–1
  cerebral 22–3
  chemotherapy 15–18, 26
  classification 12–13
  cutaneous 24
  depression 26
  distribution 11, 13–14
  fever 24
  gastro-intestinal 23
  hydronephrosis 21
  hypercalcaemia 24
  impotence 26
  infection 21–2
  infertility 26
  itching 13, 24
  long-term complications 26–7
  lymphadenopathy 19–20
  neurological syndromes 24–5
  pain 229
  palliative care 18–27
  paraneoplastic problems 24–5
  pleural effusions 23
  prognosis 14–15
  psychosexual problems 26
  radiotherapy, complications 26